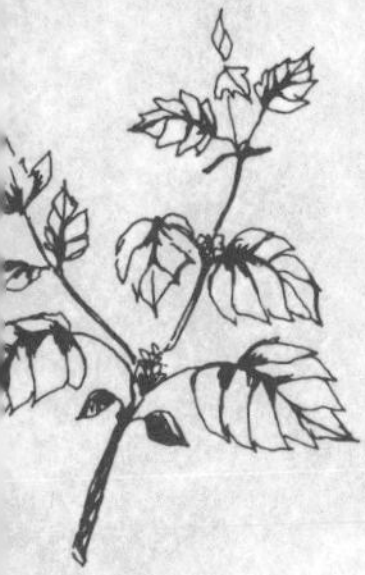

BALM

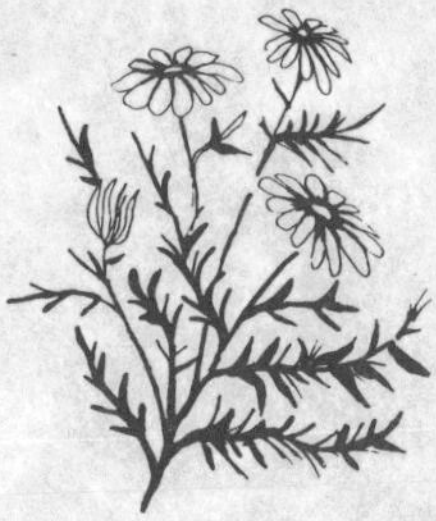

CHAMOMILE

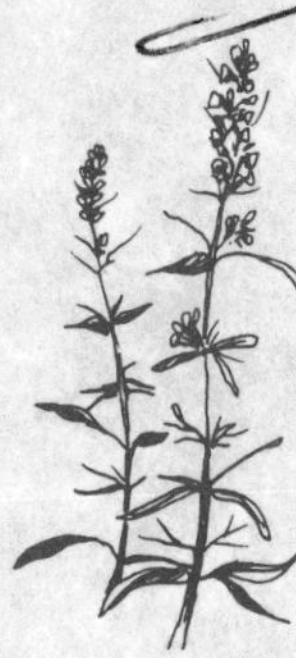

HYSSOP

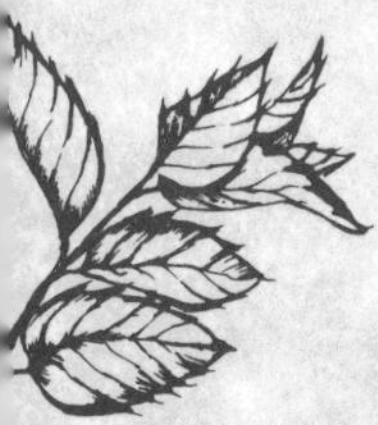

MINT

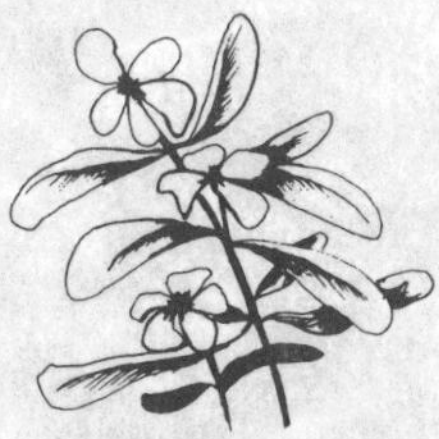

PERIWINKLE

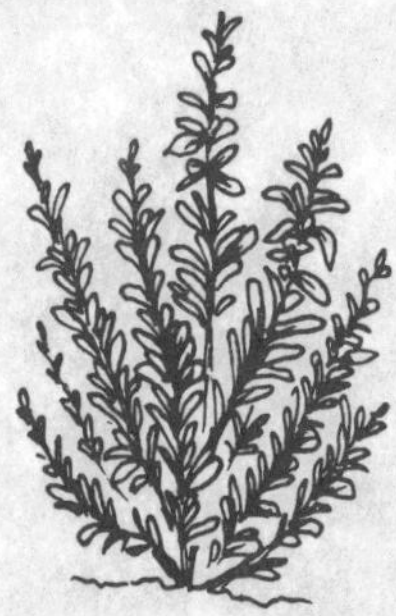

ROSEMARY

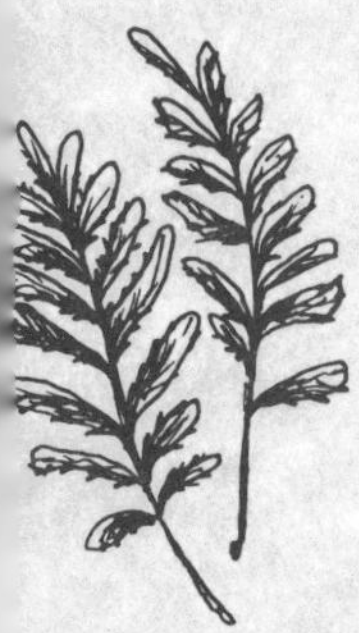

TANSY

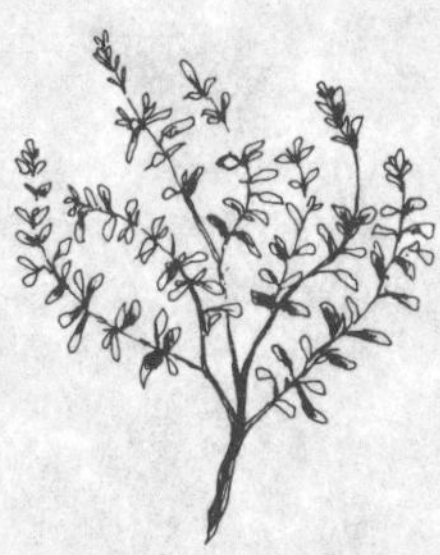

THYME

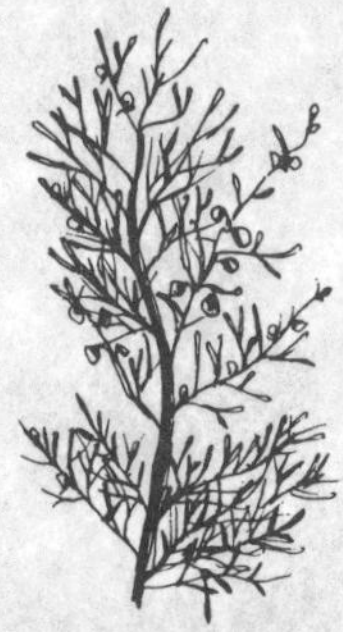

WORMWOOD

Herbs, Physicke, & Nutrition in Early America

Thomas Jefferson Treats Himself

by
John M. Holmes

Published by Loft Press, Inc.
P.O. Box 95, Fort Valley, Virginia 22652

ISBN 0-9630797-3-5
Library of Congress Catalog Card Number 97-70150

Illustrations by Sarah A. Coffman

Printed and bound in the United States of America

For Catherine and Tracey, Always.

CONTENTS

List of Illustrations vi

Preface vii

Acknowledgements ix

Chapter One
BACKGROUND
A Practice Rustic and Harsh 1

Chapter Two
DOCTORS AND DRUGS IN COLONIAL VIRGINIA
A Pious Fraud 7

Chapter Three
THOMAS JEFFERSON AND THE DOCTOR
Physicians and Vultures 21

Chapter Four
JEFFERSON AND MATERIA MEDICA
A Garden Pharmacy 39

Chapter Five
JEFFERSON ON HEALTH
I Enjoy Good Health and Spirits 67

Chapter Six
HEALTH IS THE FIRST REQUISITE
A Jefferson Legacy 85

Chapter Seven
CONCLUSIONS
A Twentieth Century Man 101

Appendix: Mr. Jefferson's Herbs 109
Bibliography 113
Index 119

Illustrations

Hyssop, *Hyssopus officinalis* 14

Rue, *Ruta graveolens* 15

Southernwood, *Artemisia abrotanum* 16

Robley Dunglison 33
Courtesy of Historical Collections and Services, The Claude Moore Health Sciences Library, The University of Virginia

Marjoram, *Marjorana hortensis* 40

Sage, *Salvia officinalis* 42

Rosemary, *Rosemarinus officinalis* 50

Chamomile, *Anthemis nobilis* 51

Balm, *Melissa officinalis* 52

Mint, *Mentha piperita* 53

Thyme, *Thymus vulgaris* 54

Lavender, *Lavandula spica* 55

Tansy, *Tanacetum vulgare* 56

Wormwood, *Artemisia absinthium* 57

Marshmallow, *Althaea officinalis* 58

Periwinkle, *Vinca minor* 59

Jefferson's Medicine Box 64
Courtesy of Monticello/Thomas Jefferson Memorial Foundation, Inc.

Thomas Jefferson, by Thomas Sully 99
Courtesy of the Thomas Jefferson Memorial Foundation; gift of Mr. and Mrs. Carl W. Smith and Mr. and Mrs. T. Eugene Worrel

PREFACE

WELL KNOWN HISTORICAL PERSONALITIES ARE REMEMBERED in terms of great events or great achievements. As a consequence, it is easy to forget how ordinary they could be. In everyday circumstances, great personalities often behaved exactly as everyday people.

Thomas Jefferson was, in many ways, the average man. He loved his family, he worried about money and he complained about government. He planted a garden, he shared visits with friends and neighbors and, occasionally, he fell ill. Viewed in this perspective, he was Everyman[1].

It is the Everyman transformation that makes Jefferson real. It endows him with flesh and blood. Here there are no pedestals, no memorials; simply a man. If Jefferson was, in many ways, the average man, then his health, health practices and use of materia medica become especially intriguing. How better to understand the everyday Jefferson? The rarefied atmosphere of Monticello could not prevent him from contracting the common cold or experiencing headaches. How did he feel? How did he treat his ailments? The achievements that made him extraordinary are a matter of record. What did he do that made him ordinary?

Understanding a commonplace phase of Jefferson's life may result in a better understanding of what is not so commonplace. Knowing how his attitudes and prejudices affected his health may, in some way, better explain his stand on more complex issues. No reader of this book will have owned a slave, built a Monticello or written a Declaration of Independence, but all

1 Everyman, a character in a fifteenth-century morality play

will have endured a cold or a headache. This shared experience alters the angle of the lens of history, creating an overlapping image of ourselves and Thomas Jefferson, and thus, allowing us the unique opportunity of experiencing the time he lived in. If timeless routine experiences can elicit empathy, then might the same be possible with the less routine ones?

This book offers a glimpse into the average world of a not-so-average man; a place where simple distance, not achievement, separated him from others. Jefferson emerges from the pages of the past into the embodiment of an everyday person. In this respect, the ordinary aspects of Jefferson's life lend an insightful perspective to the man.

Acknowledgments

NO ONE WRITES A BOOK ALONE. THE UNDERTAKING, TO BE successful, requires the support and assistance of a large number of people. Without the generous amounts of time and information given by those individuals, no successful work would ever be possible.

First and foremost, I thank my wife, Catherine, and daughter, Tracey, both of whom surrendered substantial family time without complaint and offered constant encouragement. And again, my wife, who typed every character and every correction of every copy from the first to the last page.

Sincere thanks go to the staff at the Monticello Research Center whose help and professionalism were greatly appreciated. Special thanks to Peter Hatch, Ann Lucas, Kathy Revell and Lucia C. Stanton.

An individual note of gratitude to Mary Marquis whose enthusiasm and encouragement for this work was immediate and unrestrained. Also, to Dr. Steven W. Guerrier, Associate Professor of History at James Madison University, who donated a portion of his valuable time to read and critique my work. His comments were greatly appreciated.

In addition, my appreciation for the editing done by Ann A. Hunter. Her work made the book eminently more readable.

Lastly, to my friend, Dr. Robert I. Alotta, who alone knows the whole story behind this endeavor. Bob was my teacher, editor, and overseer. Any shortcomings are mine, any strengths are his.

Thomas Jefferson Treats Himself

CHAPTER ONE

Background

A Practice Rustic and Harsh

During the early years of America's history the practice of medicine was rustic and harsh. With the advent of the heroic age of medicine and its attending purges, emetics and bleeding, many Americans developed a deep distrust of physicians. As a result, a majority of people relied on home remedies passed down through families or offered to them in self-help medical manuals.

Wealthy individuals found that money and social standing had no influence on the type of medical treatment they received. Worldly worth and community prominence could not procure better medical attention. It simply did not exist.

United in their struggle, rich and poor alike battled diseases, which they did not understand, with treatments born of desperation and ignorance. Like his contemporaries, Thomas Jefferson faced life-threatening illnesses. Characteristically, Jefferson, when faced with a problem, bore down on it with intense intellectual scrutiny. In response to the problem of maintaining health, Jefferson developed a regimen of proper diet and regular exercise and trusted in the healing powers of nature. When illness compelled him, he consulted physicians and used medicinal preparations, in many of which he had little faith.

Although Jefferson was a man obsessed with details, he seems to have had no enthusiasm for keeping a record of his illnesses and treatments. The story of his health must therefore be pieced together from his private papers and correspondence, his garden, farm and memorandum books and the large number of medical volumes in his library.

From these sources Jefferson emerges as a man highly skeptical, if not disdainful, of physicians and medicine. He made no secret of the fact that he believed the field of medicine to be grounded in theory, not science.

In accordance with many of his political and social views, Thomas Jefferson's attitudes on medicine and personal health were ahead of their time. He understood well the benefits of a proper diet, exercise and the correlation between good health and quality of life. Thomas Jefferson believed ardently that health was something to be preserved rather than restored, and that the process of preserving health establishes a lifestyle leading the individual towards realizing his full potential.

Early Americans confronted numerous problems upon their arrival in the New World. They were ill prepared for the harsh climate of their new land. The sharp cold of New England and the stifling heat and humidity of the South took their toll. Mosquitoes spread malaria and the drinking water, stagnant and putrid, teemed with lethal micro-organisms. The land was heavily forested, requiring intensive labor to clear it. Productive cultivation practices were lacking. Native inhabitants observed silently and sullenly the life or death contest between the newcomers and nature, occasionally taking an active and violent role in the struggle. Time was needed for the settlers to become acclimated to their new environment. The colonists' survival was constantly in doubt while this "seasoning" process unfolded.

Disease was an especially hideous scourge for early Americans. In addition to the malaria, smallpox, diphtheria, and cholera, many other serious diseases were a constant threat. Many who survived periods of starvation fell victim to the ravages of these various illnesses. There was no immunity among the people to these diseases. The causes, transmission and proper treatments for these carriers of death were not understood.

Those early Americans met the threat with stoicism and home remedies. Doctors, if they were available, were seldom consulted. Medical training and practice was rudimentary and primitive. These short-comings were not lost on prospective patients. As a consequence, most people lacked faith in a doctor's ability to diagnose and treat their ailments. It was an accepted fact of life that contracting a disease frequently resulted in death.

Thomas Jefferson likewise faced the dangers of illness. Although relatively free of serious health problems during his lifetime, he did suffer with some short and long term illnesses. He experienced the common cold, headaches and rheumatism. Diarrhea afflicted him for the last quarter of his life. The treatments to which he resorted, and the related topic of his general health, are the concerns of this book.

A great many biographers and historians have devoted years to researching and writing about Jefferson's life. Thousands of books and articles are available which deal with nearly every aspect of his day-to-day existence. However, no scholar has yet devoted time or energy to Jefferson's use of materia medica.

Earliest among the biographers was Henry Randall, who, with the assistance of members of Jefferson's family, wrote the first extensive life of Thomas Jefferson.[1] Randall, an admirer of Jefferson, produced a work that portrays him as a man who possessed few, if any, flaws. Following Randall, more serious minded scholars took their turns at understanding the Man from Monticello. Dumas Malone wrote a multi-volumed work[2] which ranks as one of the best studies done to date. Malone, devoting more than thirty years to his project, turned out an even-handed evaluation of Jefferson. Merrill Peterson, another Jefferson scholar, in his work, *Thomas Jefferson: Writings*, provides historians with a selection of informative texts accompanied by Peterson's insightful notes. Other historians have concentrated on singular aspects of Jefferson's life.

John Chester Miller's, *The Wolf by the Ears,* is a candid and thought provoking work on Jefferson and slavery. Fawn Brodie, in her controversial work, *Thomas Jefferson: An Intimate Biography,* details the private side of Jefferson's life, focusing on the Sally Hemings question.

Jefferson's granddaughter, Sarah Jefferson Randolph, compiled an intimate family view of Jefferson as husband, father and grandfather. *The Domestic Life of Thomas Jefferson* is a tribute to a man who loved well and was well loved in return.

Collaboration by pairs of historians has yielded volumes rich in detailed information. James A. Bear, Jr., and Edwin Betts; Adrienne Koch and William Peden have produced well edited and highly readable compilations of Jefferson's writings and correspondence. Their works, respectively, *The Family*

1 Randall, Henry S. *The Life of Thomas Jefferson.* 3 vols. New York: Derby & Jackson, 1858.

2 Malone, Dumas. *Jefferson and His Time.* 6 vols. Boston: Little, Brown and Company, 1948.

Letters of Thomas Jefferson and *The Life and Selected Writings of Thomas Jefferson,* reveal the personal side of Jefferson and are invaluable sources for Jefferson scholars.

At Princeton University the editing of thousands of pages of Jefferson's papers has been ongoing for several years. Today, John Catanzariti heads this monumental task. When completed the work may easily approach fifty or more volumes in length.

For the present book, significant primary source materials were *Thomas Jefferson's Garden Book*, edited by Edwin Betts and *Jefferson's Memorandum Books: Accounts, with Legal Records and Miscellany, 1767-1826,* edited by James A. Bear, Jr., and Lucia C. Stanton (forthcoming). Both supplied detailed insights into Jefferson's involvement with the operation of Monticello and personal expenditures.

As mentioned previously, despite the close scrutiny to which Jefferson and his life have been subjected, one area has remained untouched. The topic of Jefferson's medicinal practices has been ignored by historical scholars. So too, his attitudes towards diet and exercise have never been formally examined. Jefferson stood more or less alone with his views of medicine and health care. While some of his contemporaries shared similar attitudes, none professed the consistent and candid opposition to medical practices and physicians expressed by Jefferson. Benjamin Franklin's health habits paralleled Jefferson's in terms of exercise and moderation but diverged at Franklin's use of purges and strict reliance on the doctor. George Washington made frequent use of bleeding, a procedure rejected by Jefferson, and habitually purchased substantial amounts of medicine, something Jefferson did not do. John Adams admitted to enjoying tobacco for more than fifty years, whereas Jefferson, apparently convinced of its detrimental health effects, never used it during his lifetime.

Thomas Jefferson was a man of many dimensions. This

book reveals yet another of them. It marks only the beginning of an effort to uncover and identify the total story of Thomas Jefferson's health and use of medicines. Its purpose is to provide one more window through which we may view the fascinating life of this remarkable man.

CHAPTER TWO

Doctors and Drugs in Colonial Virginia

A Pious Fraud

THE HEAVILY FORESTED LAND IN VIRGINIA TO WHICH the early English settlers came was forbidding and dangerous. It offered them, at best, a tenuous existence where only the strongest would survive. Escaping death would require all the resolve, skill and faith that they could muster.

Native inhabitants, Indians, eyed these strangers cautiously from the forest's edge. The newcomers appeared strangely clothed and carried odd looking weapons. The Indians, wary of the light-skinned arrivals, avoided them. After a time, however, the plight of the aliens moved the Indians. Spurred on by a generosity of spirit, they cast aside their caution and sympathetically offered the colonists assistance. Perhaps unwittingly, but still no less genuinely, by their actions the Indians had issued a moral challenge. Time and circumstances would determine the colonists' response.

The many difficulties that the colonists confronted, the Indians had long before faced and overcome. Shelter, food and medicine, basics for survival, they had much earlier learned to obtain from the land. Adapting to nature, the Indians found out how to work with her, not against her. The vast forest and its abundant game provided them with their first two necessities: shelter and food. Knowledge of medicine, however, was acquired by chance, and trial and error. That knowledge, highly valued, was carefully handed down from generation to generation. Medicine men tutored protegees in the mysteries of healing. This assured that ritual actions and herbal medicines would be retained when the older men died. The oral passing of information from generation to generation ran the inherent risk of the loss of meaningful facts. But in the absence of a true written language, and possessed of a strong desire for secrecy, Indians had to rely on verbal transmission.

Although it is risky to generalize about the medicinal habits of Indians it can be stated that for all of them, "their materia medica was almost exclusively herbal."[1] Almost solely, plants supplied all of the therapeutic needs of the Indian peoples. They used the powdered roots of skunk cabbage for asthma, soaproot for dandruff and a tonic of boiled wild mint for nausea.[2] A great many other plants, as well, were highly valued by the Indians for their medicinal benefits.

It was not unusual for diverse tribes to employ the same plant in altogether different ways. For instance,

> the handsome blue flag (*Iris versicolor*) was cultivated by the Creek Indians as a cathartic; the Albany Indians used its root crushed as a poultice for leg-ulcers; the Meskwakis made a decoction of the roots for colds and lung problems; the Ojibwa considered it an emetic; and the Penobscots believed it was a complete panacea, thought by some to be their most treasured medicine.[3]

---

1 Barbara Griggs, *Green Pharmacy* (Rochester, Vermont: Healing Arts Press, 1991), p. 101.

2 Benjamin Capps, *The Indians* (New York: Time-Life Books, 1976), p. 139.

3 Barbara Griggs, *Green Pharmacy* (Rochester, Vermont: Healing Arts Press, 1991), p. 101.

The Indians' extensive knowledge of botanical medicines formed the basis of a later quest by the colonists for other remedies native to their new homeland.

In addition to using plant medicines the Indians also practiced bloodletting. Bleeding by Indians served the same purpose as bleeding by doctors in Europe: to allow poisonous material to be removed from the body. The Indian doctor "tried to draw out blood and other matter from the sick or wounded person. [Thus] releasing the ill humor from a painful joint or limb . . . . "[4]

Indian and European medicine were similar as well in the use of heat and steam for sweating. John Smith wrote of one such treatment describing the procedure for constructing an air-tight enclosure and having a fire built within it. The patient suffering from "dropsies, swellings, aches, and such like diseases" entered and began the therapy.[5] A contemporary of Smith's noted matter-of-factly that the patient then "either recovers, or gives up the ghost."[6]

Another exception to the use of plants as medicine was a particular variety of clay employed by the Indians in Virginia. They, according to a colonist, ". . . eate it for physicke, alleaging that it cureth the sicknesse and paine of the belly."[7] Probably the porous clay acted in a fashion similar to an antacid thus relieving indigestion and flatulence.

Disease compounded for the colonists, as it did for the Indians, the harsh realities of existence. At any moment serious illness could strike a colonial family and, in the early years especially, frequently did. This threat was exacerbated by the

---

4 Thomas P. Hughes, *Medicine in Virginia, 1607–1699* (Williamsburg, Virginia: Va. 350th Anniv. Celebration Corp., 1957), p. 9.

5 Ibid., p. 10.

6 Ibid.

7 Ibid., p. 11.

colonists' inability to cultivate crops, which would have supplied them with better food, and a slow acclimation to their new environment. Both predicaments were serious problems which brought on a weakened physical state. This infirmity heightened their susceptibility to illness and decreased the odds for their survival. In addition, the hot and humid summers of the Virginia colony provided a fertile breeding ground for a variety of new diseases.

The small number of medical men who accompanied the early settlers were poorly trained and knew only slightly more about the diseases and treatments than did their patients. They succumbed to these ailments as readily as the settlers themselves. When abandoned through death by their "healers," and essentially ignorant of the diseases, the colonists responded to sickness in the only way they could. In these lonely and frightening circumstances, self-medication was their only recourse.

Having few doctors in the colony was of limited consequence. As the population expanded into the countryside, many people were physically too distant from a physician for practical consultation. Most physicians practiced near the sea coast in the larger towns. Few, if any, trekked into the backwoods. Those who did venture into the wilderness were usually received with more suspicion than appreciation. In such cases "a preference for self-care, high fees and unreliable cures led colonial Virginians to [generally avoid] their physicians. . . ."[8] Most early doctors had been trained abroad, there being no medical school in Virginia or any other colony until the late eighteenth century (the first opened in Philadelphia in 1765). Many later practitioners simply studied medicine at the elbow of a practicing physician.[9] It was wholly too expensive, and the

8 Todd L. Savitt, *Fevers, Agues, and Cures* (Richmond, Virginia: Virginia Historical Society, 1990), p. 29.

dangers of a sea crossing too frightful, for most parents to send their sons to Europe for medical training. But prospective patients tended to be wary of the treatment, the expense, and the doctor himself, whether he was trained abroad formally or through apprenticeship to a local physician.

In western Virginia many settlers of varied nationalities chose the mountain and valley region. Scotch, German and Scotch-Irish immigrants claimed ownership of land which for centuries had been tribal home to the Indians. Into this rugged and rich country they "brought a different language and culture and some different medical folkways to Virginia."[10] These settlers were bred from hardy stock and were taught self-reliance during their youth. Consequently, they gravitated towards self-treatment and natural remedies. It was not in their character to succumb to every ache and pain. Their first inclination when illness struck was to reach for a tonic and then get on with work.

This tendency to rely on self-care and home remedies, combined with a skepticism of physicians, resulted in settlers becoming their own doctors. For them, it seemed in keeping with the American spirit that people should assume responsibility for their own physical well-being. When you broke the land with your own hands, relied on your own wits to survive and took no man's counsel to decide your fate, then you also took upon yourself the right and responsibility to safeguard and administer your own health.

The taming of America was not for the faint of heart. It required sinewy arms and calloused hands and a willingness to fight, if it came to that, for "me and mine." The rugged and raw environment produced a fiercely independent breed of man,

---

9 Ibid., p. 29.

10 Ibid., p. 31.

who would guard his right to dictate his health care as he would guard any other personal possession.

Exercising this particular right owed as much to doubt about doctors as it did to personal independence. People believed, with good reason, that in most, if not all cases, the doctor's cure was worse than the illness. Treatments were harsh and caused great misery. Bleeding, purging and emetics were three severe courses of action almost always employed by early doctors. The ensuing loss of blood and upheaval of the alimentary system often had disastrous effects. As one author noted of early physicians, "until well into the 19th Century dogmas were so rigid, theories so doctrinaire, hands and instruments so germ-ridden, and 'remedies' so enervating that the learned doctor often did less to cure than to kill the patient."[11] The struggle for survival was difficult enough without a doctor tipping the scales against you.

The diseases faced by early settlers were lethal. Malaria, typhoid and diphtheria, among others, were widespread in colonial Virginia. These names are familiar to contemporary readers. Colonists, however, called them intermittent fever (malaria), slow fever (typhoid), and putrid sore throat or rotten Quinsy (diphtheria).[12]

The three diseases killed, each in its own relentless way. Intermittent fever, spread by the bite of the anopheles mosquito, was a bane to every settler. (Virginia's Tidewater area was an ideal breeding ground for the mosquito.) Characterized by periodic attacks of chills and fever, malaria held the colonies in a mortal grip until the discovery of Peruvian Bark (quinine) curtailed its fearsome assault. Outbreaks of slow fever, an

---

11 Daniel J. Boorstin, *The Americans: The Colonial Experience* (New York: Vintage Books, 1958), p. 214.

12 Harold B. Gill, Jr., *The Apothecary in Colonial Virginia* (Williamsburg, Virginia: Colonial Williamsburg Foundation, 1972), p. 96.

infection of the digestive system caused by a bacterium, were the result of the colonists drinking contaminated water. The belief that all fresh water was safe to drink encouraged the spread of typhoid and had deadly consequences for many unfortunates. Finally, putrid sore throat or rotten Quinsy, an acute highly contagious infection that attacks the throat of the victim, generally resulted in a quick death by heart failure or asphyxiation. Diphtheria struck with unrelenting finality.

Physicians treated these illnesses with extreme methods and medications. Ipecac and senna are typical of the botanical medicines they used to induce vomiting and promote evacuation of the bowels; cupping, a method of extracting blood, quite frequently preceded or followed the medicine. While a few patients quietly accepted these traditional methods of treatment, a large number failed to see any good attached to them and sought out alternatives.

Virginians believed that when sick, their bodies' systems were out of balance. A cure meant reestablishing equilibrium. For centuries Europeans had relied on herbs and woodland plants for this restoration, the idea being "to restore the natural balance of the body with its environment . . . by taking medicines that promote recovery of that balance."[13] To retrieve this natural balance patients used vegetable medicines, prepared according to herbals and old family recipes. In addition, they might, on occasion, use patented botanical medications purchased from an apothecary.

Nicholas Culpeper, in his work, *Culpeper's Complete Herbal,* discussed several ways of treating common illnesses. For agues (fevers) such as those associated with malaria he suggested the use of chamomile and dandelion; for flux (diarrhea)

---

13 Todd L. Savitt, *Fevers, Agues and Cures* (Richmond, Virginia: Virginia Historical Society, 1990), p. 37.

like that accompanying typhoid he recommended basil and rhubarb; and, for throat ailments, such as rotten Quinsy, he advised the use of balm and hyssop.[14] If patients opted for medicine from the apothecary they might be sold mixtures composed of a large number of ingredients—veritable hodgepodges—with equally generous claims for effectiveness (patients needed to feel that they were getting their money's worth). Many of these compounds were sold as cure-all medicines. One such remedy, "rudbeckia (*Echinacea angustifolia*)," was purported to cure malaria, typhoid, diphtheria and, should the need arise, rabies as well.[15]

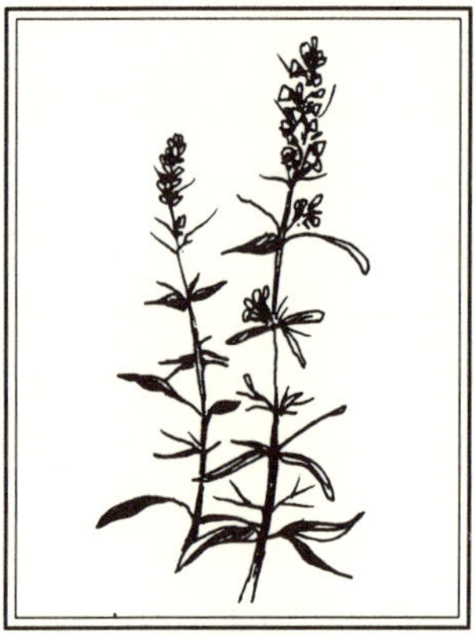

Hyssop
Hyssopus officinalis

In keeping with their propensity for self-treatment, and following their European heritage, colonists grew herbs and collected wild plants for use as medicine. Herbs such as rue, chamomile and lavender were grown in a family's small herb garden and supplemented with such forest plants as sassafras, ginseng and lobelia. From these herbs and plants settlers produced concoctions, decoctions, poultices and other medicinal compositions to treat the sick. Undoubtedly, many of these traditional remedies worked as well or better than expensive patent medicines. At the same time they were a bane to physicians, for successful treatment with them bolstered the colonists' belief that they could do well without the doctor. In a more important sense, however, these successes contributed to a better understanding of how to fight the onslaught of disease.

---

14 Nicholas Culpeper, *Culpeper's Complete Herbal* (London: W. Foulsham & Co., Ltd., n.d.), 37–293 passim.

15 Barbara Griggs, *Green Pharmacy* (Rochester, Vermont: Healing Arts Press, 1991),p. 265.

In larger Virginia gardens, like Thomas Jefferson's at Monticello, a wider variety of herbs was grown. More herbs represented a greater capacity for treating illnesses. At Monticello, tansy, wormwood, lavender, chamomile, rue, southernwood and periwinkle were just a few of the herbs grown and used medicinally.[16] For therapeutic use it was necessary that each herb be processed in a prescribed manner and administered properly for specific diseases. *Culpeper's Complete Herbal*, and other similar pharmacopoeias provided advice on how to prepare and use the herbs. For instance, Culpeper's book advised that for tansy, "the leaves only are used, and are astringent and vulnerary, good to stop all kinds of fluxes and preternatural evacuations, to dissolve congealed blood, [and] to help those who are bruised by falls."[17] For rue, Culpeper stated:

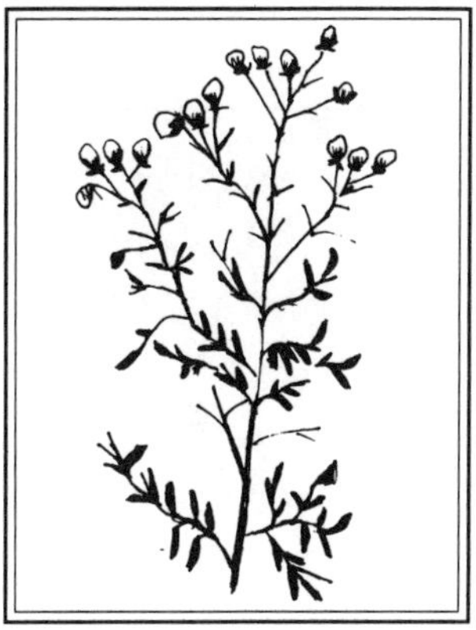

Rue
Ruta graveloens

> The seed taken in wine, is an antidote against all dangerous medicines or deadly poisons. A decoction made with some dried dill-leaves and flowers, . . . if drunk, helps the pains of the chest and sides, coughs and hardness of breathing, inflammations of the lungs and the tormenting pains of the sciatica and the joints . . .[18]

Southernwood, Culpeper's herbal claimed, is useful for "those that are troubled with cramps or convulsions . . . [and] it removes pimples."[19] As these examples point out, it was not unusual for an herb

---

16 Edwin Morris Betts, *Thomas Jefferson's Garden Book* (Lancaster, Pennsylvania: Lancaster Press, Inc., 1944), p. 208.

17 Nicholas Culpeper, *Culpeper's Complete Herbal* (London: W. Foulsham & Co., Ltd., n.d.), p. 361.

18 Ibid., p. 304.

19 Ibid., p. 341.

to be characterized as having the capacity for easing the symptoms of, or curing, many different health problems.

As mentioned earlier, plants as well as herbs played an important role in the medicaments employed by early Virginians. For years, beginning with the earliest Virginia settlements doctors and interested lay persons scoured Virginia's forests looking for plants possessing medicinal value. In many instances their efforts were successful. In 1788, for example, William Cabell recorded in his diary that a decoction made from persimmon with added ingredients produced an excellent medication for a "wound or old ulcer [skin eruption]."[20] Also, *Medical Botany*, a work by Walter Lewis, states that the roots of the common wild dandelion were found to be an effective treatment for chronic liver diseases.[21] Thomas Jefferson in his *Notes on the State of Virginia*, written in 1781, listed a large number of native Virginia plants which he believed warranted attention for their medicinal value. Among these were Palma christi (Ricinus), Euphorbia Ipecacuanhae (ipecac), Virginia snake-root, Ginseng and Indian physic.[22] Indian physic had long been popular with Virginians as an emetic. William Byrd, of Virginia, recorded in his diary that he found it "an excellent vomit."[23]

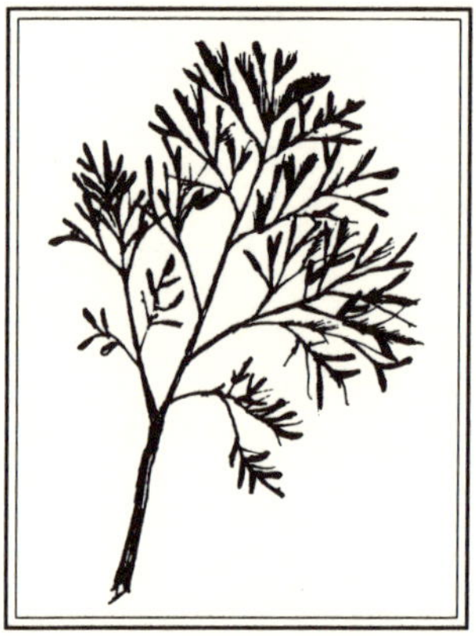

Southernwood
Artemisia abrotanum

The various herbs and plants available provided the early

20 Harold B. Gill, Jr., *The Apothecary in Colonial Virginia* (Williamsburg, Virginia: Colonial Williamsburg Foundation, 1972), pp. 43–44.

21 Walter H. Lewis, *Medical Botany* (New York: John Wiley & Sons, 1977), p. 289.

22 Edwin Morris Betts, *Thomas Jefferson's Garden Book* (Lancaster, Pennsylvania: Lancaster Press, Inc., 1944), pp. 644–655.

23 Barbara Griggs, *Green Pharmacy* (Rochester, Vermont: Healing Arts Press, 1981), p. 140.

colonists with what they believed to be potent weapons against a formidable enemy. Trusting in botanical preparations helped reassure them when facing an illness and gave them an excuse to avoid the dreaded physician. Although on the whole physicians were well intentioned, most often the patient's needs exceeded the doctor's abilities. Certainly most physicians did their best. Quite regularly, however, their best was not good enough. Practicing with only a superficial understanding of the human body, their efforts amounted to little more than sophisticated quackery. As alluded to earlier, many physicians were trained through apprenticeship; consequently, any lack of learning carried over from doctor to apprentice.[24] Thus, a seriously flawed system perpetuated itself.

The prospect of bleeding was dreaded by many patients. Bloodletting, probably as old as medicine itself, was considered necessary by early physicians to bring about healing. Unfortunately, most doctors did not have the good sense to know when enough was enough. Many a miserable victim was bled white by the good doctor in the belief that he was saving a life. The treatment of George Washington during his final illness is an excellent example of this. Washington's attending physicians "extracted over four pints of [his] blood."[25] In all probability, the loss of that much blood contributed directly to his death.

Bleeding had as one of its major proponents "Dr. Benjamin Rush [who] was largely responsible for its continued popularity in nineteenth-century America."[26] Dr. Rush, a renowned Philadelphia physician, signer of the Declaration of Independence and close friend of Thomas Jefferson, lacked any aware-

---

24 Todd L. Savitt, *Fevers, Agues and Cures* (Richmond, Virginia: Virginia Historical Society, 1990), p. 56.

25 J. Dwyer and D. Rattray, eds., *Magic and Medicine of Plants* (Pleasantville, New York: Reader's Digest Association, Inc., 1993), p. 67.

26 Ibid., p. 39.

ness that the body could not produce blood as quickly as performing bleeding might remove it. In fact, Rush believed it almost impossible to bleed a patient to death. In a letter to Dr. Thomas Cooper, dated October 7, 1814, Jefferson wrote, "in his theory of bleeding . . ., I was ever opposed to my friend Rush, whom I greatly loved; but who had done much harm, in the sincerest persuasion that he was preserving life and happiness to all around him."[27]

It was partly because of excesses like Rush's that a great many colonists chose to consult doctors only as a final resort, after home remedies had failed to produce satisfactory results. Even at this point, many sufferers preferred to place their fate in the "hands of God" rather than the "grasp of the doctor." It is fair to say that colonial physicians, as Barbara Griggs has pointed out, "had an appallingly bad reputation: if you could save a friend from falling into the clutches of the medical profession by passing on some tried and trusted family recipe for his disorder, you would be rendering him a service indeed."[28]

Thomas Jefferson was gravely disturbed by the short-comings of physicians and medicine. Within his correspondence are many statements that reflect his uneasy feelings about the practitioners and the practice. Because of his unease, Jefferson determined to preserve the good health he already enjoyed rather than having to restore any of that health he might otherwise lose. To that end, Jefferson incorporated a number of sound health measures into his daily routine. He ate little red meat, but large amounts of vegetables; he drank only weak wines and he refused to use tobacco. He exercised each day, generally by riding horseback or taking brisk walks. These mea-

---

27 John M. Dorsey, M.D., ed., *The Jefferson—Dunglison Letters* (Charlottesville, Virginia: University of Virginia Press, 1960), p. 105.

28 Barbara Griggs, *Green Pharmacy* (Rochester, Vermont: Healing Arts Press, 1991), p. 109.

sures which today are viewed as sensible health practices were not widely perceived as such in Jefferson's day. Jefferson, however, believed in them and not the doctor. He therefore incorporated them into his lifestyle.

Not all of Jefferson's peers shared his prejudices against doctors, heroic medicine or even tobacco. George Washington, John Marshall and John Adams all left records and correspondence indicating their willingness to seek the services of physicians. And, for Washington at least, the use of severe medical treatments was not unusual. Adams, the master diarist, recorded his early introduction to tobacco and his continued use of it for almost sixty years.[29] Ironically, though they died the same day, Adams, the tobacco user, outlived Jefferson, who shunned it, by eight years.

While they had no qualms about consulting a doctor, George Washington and John Marshall also self-medicated using both commercial preparations and medicines produced at home. Washington regularly ordered large quantities of common and patented medicines for delivery to Mount Vernon. And, Marshall, this time favoring domestic medicine, advised his son that the boy's mother wished him to use sassafras twigs soaked in water to produce a "jelly" with which to treat inflammation of the eye.[30]

Thomas Jefferson was one of only a small number of prominent early Americans who seemed to value and practice health maintenance. He took those steps that he believed would keep him healthy and fit. When ill, he would occasionally consult a physician. As often as possible, however, he preferred to rely on the recuperative powers of nature.

---

29 L. H. Butterfield, ed., *Diary and Autobiography of John Adams* (Cambridge, Massachusetts: Belknap Press of Harvard Univ., 1961), p. 13.

30 Todd L. Savitt, *Fevers, Agues and Cures* (Richmond, Virginia: Virginia Historical Society, 1990), pp. 33–37.

Safe-guarding his health and being in command of his health care were responsibilities Thomas Jefferson took seriously and fully intended to act upon.

CHAPTER THREE

Jefferson and the Doctor

Physicians And Vultures

IN 1824 DR. ROBLEY DUNGLISON LEFT HIS OBSTETRIC practice in London to bring his advanced medical theories to Mr. Jefferson's new University in Charlottesville[1]. Inevitably, he found himself in attendance upon the former president. The last physician to treat Thomas Jefferson, Dr. Dunglison, in his *Personal Memoranda,* refers to a comment that perfectly illustrates Jefferson's attitude towards physicians. It seems that Jefferson, while in the presence of a Dr. Everett, observed "that whenever he saw three physicians together, he looked up to discover whether there was not a turkey buzzard in the neighborhood."[2] Dr. Dunglison explained that while he personally found the story humorous, Dr. Everett was, at the time, somewhat put out by it.

1 The University of Virginia, chartered in 1819, opened in 1825.

2 John M. Dorsey, M.D., ed., *The Jefferson-Dunglison Letters* (Charlottesville, Virginia: University of Virginia Press, 1960), p. 105.

Jefferson had little faith in physicians and the practice of medicine. In a letter to William Green Munford, written in 1799, Jefferson declared, "The state of medicine is worse than that of total ignorance."[3] Jefferson could not have made his position more clear.

Jefferson believed in the infallibility of nature. He reasoned that nature, if left alone, would restore the natural balance which had been undone by disease. Doctors, he felt, interfered with this restorative process. Their slavish devotion to purging, emetics and bleeding served only to torment the patient. In *Notes on the State of Virginia,* Jefferson complained of hospitals where "the sick, the dying and the dead are crammed together in the same rooms, and often in the same beds" and that doctors most often failed to save them.[4] However, among people eschewing the physician and self-treating at home "nature and kind nursing save a much greater proportion . . . and with less abuse."[5] This short sentence summarizes Jefferson's stance on medicine. Nature was a more reliable and gentler healer than any doctor. When all was said and done, Jefferson "trusted most *vis medicatrix naturae.*"[6]

In a later expression of this same feeling Jefferson, in a letter to Dr. Caspar Wistar dated June 21, 1807, remarked, "she [nature] brings on a crisis, by stools, vomiting, sweat, urine, expectoration, bleeding, and [etc.], which, for the most part ends in the restoration of healthy action."[7] Physicians, on the

---

3 Merrill D. Peterson, *Thomas Jefferson: Writings* (New York: The Library of America, 1984), p. 1065.

4 A. Koch and W. Peden, eds., *The Life and Selected Writings of Thomas Jefferson* (New York: Random House, 1993), p. 233.

5 Ibid.

6 Harry Bloch, M.D., "Thomas Jefferson 1743 to 1826," *N.Y. State Journal of Medicine* Vol. 72 (December 15, 1972): p. 3030.

7 Merrill D. Peterson, *Thomas Jefferson: Writings* (New York: The Library of America, 1984), pp. 1182–1183.

other hand, he told Wistar, were a danger to life itself. "I believe we may safely affirm, that the inexperienced and presumptuous band of medical tyros let loose upon the world," he wrote, "destroys more of human life in one year, than all the Robinhoods, Cartouches, and Macheaths do in a century."[8] Here again, he pronounced his faith in nature's healing power and his scorn for then existent medicine. Clearly, in Jefferson's mind, the Grim Reaper bore a sickle in one hand and a black medical bag in the other.

Jefferson was convinced of the body's ability to heal itself. Any interference with this process he found objectionable. Even when calling in a physician could not be avoided, Jefferson refused radical treatment. So-called "heroic medicine" he held to be worse than any disease. And, he was also on the lookout to avoid what he believed to be many a doctor's tendency to employ another form of quackery. "One of the most successful physicians I have ever known," Jefferson wrote, "has assured me, that he used more bread pills, drops of colored water, and powders of hickory ashes, than all other medicines put together."[9] This, Jefferson was convinced, constituted the worst type of professional fraud. More to the point, the use of "sugar pills" insulted his intelligence. He made no allowance for the placebo effect.

In general, traditional therapy involved the use of "fashionable treatments" which he found offensive, the only bright spot being that "sometimes [patients] get well in spite of the medicine."[10] Jefferson perceived that medicine was practiced as an art, not a science: an art, he believed, where human exertions countered the efforts of nature to heal, not a science

---

8 Ibid.

9 A. Koch and W. Peden, eds., *The Life and Selected Writings of Thomas Jefferson* (New York: Random House, 1993), p. 534.

10 Ibid., p. 535.

where study and experience would lead to knowledge which could then be applied methodically.

Resentment, and worse, was often directed at colonial doctors. Robert Beverley, of Virginia, in 1705 observed that the planters "have the happiness to have very few Doctors, and those such as make use only of simple Remedies."[11] Too often physicians proved by their ineptness that they were more to be feared than respected. It was no wonder. As Daniel J. Boorstin has observed, "the common medical treatments here did not cure any more effectively than those administered in the Old World" and here, as well, doctors believed illnesses to be the result of a "maladjustment of the general 'system' of the body [or] disorder in the 'humors' [or] disturbance of the bodily 'tension' " and even cruder causes.[12] Losing family members was traumatic. That they might have been lost to the incompetence of a physician could only compound the family's grief. Such losses were compelling inducements to self-care.

Another consideration, if one was needed, constraining patients from consulting physicians was the doctor's misplaced tendency towards high fees. As early as 1639 the law attempted to soften the "immoderate and excessive rates and prices exacted by practitioners in physic and churgery."[13] As a result, the rates were set and applied to two categories of surgeons, those who learned medicine by apprenticeship and those who studied at a university. Apprenticeship trained surgeons could charge up to five shillings for a visit in town or within a five-mile radius while university-trained surgeons could charge up to ten shillings within the same area.[14] Simply put, university training

11 Daniel J. Boorstin, *The Americans: The Colonial Experience* (New York: Vintage Books, 1958), p. 210.

12 Ibid., p. 212.

13 Todd L. Savitt, *Fevers, Agues and Cures* (Richmond, Virginia: Virginia Historical Society, 1990), p. 29.

was esteemed twice as worthwhile as on-the-job training. For many Virginians, these fees represented an expenditure that they could ill afford. No matter, however, for the growing preference for home care, coupled with a lack of accessibility to doctors, essentially made the fees irrelevant.

Jefferson, who could afford the physician's fee, would allow himself to call in a doctor when he felt that he was suffering from more than a common illness. For all his bluster against the medical profession he was willing to hedge his bets. On one occasion, Jefferson was suffering from a skin rash. Dr. Dunglison, then Jefferson's personal physician, prescribed the use of a mercury ointment to quell the affliction. A disagreeable salivation, brought on by the mercury entering his system, sharply annoyed Jefferson. He complained of this unpleasant side effect to an acquaintance, whereupon the man replied, "Mr. Jefferson, you are the last man in the world, from your hatred of physic, whom I would have expected any excess in taking physic." Jefferson responded, "Yes, but I would rather have the devil than the itch."[15] Jefferson was practical. Experiencing the torment of an incessant itch impelled him to try just about anything, including the despised doctor and his medicine.

In the years before the arrival of Dunglison, Jefferson had used the services of several other doctors. His close friend, Benjamin Rush, and George Gilmer, Jr., a neighbor, both treated Jefferson on different occasions. Jefferson seemed, however, to develop a particular fondness for Dunglison. Although, as noted, Jefferson was annoyed by Dunglison's remedy, he and the doctor were destined to develop a reciprocating relationship of trust, respect and admiration. Jefferson

14 Thomas K. Ford, *The Apothecary in Eighteenth-Century Williamsburg* (Williamsburg, Virginia: Colonial Williamsburg, 1987), p. 7.

15 John M. Dorsey, M.D., ed., *The Jefferson-Dunglison Letters* (Charlottesville, Virginia: University of Virginia Press, 1960), p. 87.

became so pleased, in fact, with Dunglison's abilities that he wrote him, " . . . nature is preferable to an unskilled [physician]. I had therefore made up my mind to trust to her altogether, until your arrival gave me better prospects."[16]

The occasional use of medications was not the only type of treatment employed at various times by Jefferson. Another that he felt held promise was hot mineral baths. While in France in 1787, having succeeded Benjamin Franklin as Minister to the French Court, he wrote his daughter, Martha, that he had traveled to Aix-en-Provence, from Paris, to seek relief from a weakness in his hand. "It [the journey] was undertaken with the hope," he wrote, "that the mineral waters of this place might restore strength to my wrist."[17] Years later, during the summer of 1818, Jefferson again sought treatment in natural warm baths and again, his discomfort involved a joint. On August 7, he wrote Martha from Warm Springs, Virginia, "An attack of rheumatism in the knee yesterday . . . affects my walking. I have tried once to-day the delicious bath and shall do it twice a day hereafter."[18] Within a week's time, having soaked in the warm waters several times a day, Jefferson's condition improved and he thought his rheumatism eliminated. In the same letter to Martha, he told her, "I . . . presume the seeds of my rheumatism eradicated . . . I believe I shall yield to the general advice of a three weeks course."[19] However, slightly more than a month later, during the second week of September, Jefferson wrote his grandson, Francis Wayles Eppes, from Monticello, "I am lately returned from the warm springs with my health entirely prostrated by the use of the waters. They

---

16 Ibid., p. 12.

17 E. Betts and J. Bear, Jr., eds., *The Family Letters of Thomas Jefferson* (Columbia, Missouri: University of Missouri Press, 1966), p. 34.

18 Ibid., p. 424.

19 Ibid., p. 425.

produced an imposthume [abscess] and eruptions [boils] . . . ."[20] There is no evidence that Jefferson ever again sought to use mineral baths for therapy. Nature, on this occasion, had failed him.

Natural mineral baths had been popular among the social elite for several centuries. They believed that baths had the power to cure almost anything. A planter wrote his wife extolling the virtues of bathing in the waters. With his tongue planted firmly in his cheek, he declared that the waters would cure, "Yellow jaundice, white swelling, blue devils and black plague, scarlet fever, yellow fever, spotted fever and fever of every kind and colour. Hydrocephales, Hydorthoras, Hydrocele, Hydorphobia, Hypochondria and Hypocrisy, Dispepsia, Diabetes, and die-of-anything, Gout and Grogging."[21]

Although the planter was making light of the cure-all reputation of the baths, his litany of diseases gives a glimpse of the curative powers attributed to them. His lengthy list also suggests the large number of people who sought relief from their ills by immersing themselves in these naturally heated pools.

It is easy to understand the appeal of the baths to Jefferson. To him, they represented an extension of the restorative ability of nature. Throughout his life, he possessed a reverential attitude towards the natural processes he saw unfolding around him. The healing process was one, he believed, that he might experience for himself. Soaking in a mineral bath, he judged, would allow nature the opportunity to resolve his problems of a weak joint and rheumatism. Then there was his insatiable curiosity. Possessed of a keen power of observation and a need to understand, Jefferson allowed nothing to escape his scientific

---

20 Ibid., p. 427.

21 Catherine Clinton, *The Plantation Mistress* (New York: Pantheon Books, 1982), p. 149.

scrutiny. He strove at all times to unravel the mysteries of the world around him.

Binding proof of Jefferson's fascination with nature is contained in his *Garden Book.* The thousands of entries in this book testify to Jefferson's preoccupation with plants and their growing patterns. How many times had he witnessed the ability of plants to survive the loss of leaves, a damaged stem or even a cutting? Nature's remarkable capacity to heal and endure played out before him time and again. This marvelous recuperative ability inspired Jefferson's recognition of nature as preeminent physician. Because nature was continually healing herself would she not also heal Man? He was, after all, her finest effort.

On the occasions that Thomas Jefferson resided at Monticello, healing was facilitated by the use of herbs and plants. He cultivated more than a dozen herbs along with a number of other plants that, like the herbs, held medicinal properties. The ostensible benefits were covered in detail within the pharmacopoeias lining his library shelves. The snipping of some leaves along with a few glances at a page were all that was necessary to produce a variety of botanical remedies.

Despite Jefferson's prejudiced feelings towards the field of medicine, he willingly partook of some medications. During his lifetime Jefferson ingested calomel, jalap, rhubarb, quinine, magnesia and laudanum. This was no lapse of faith in nature's healing power; rather it was Jefferson's concession that some medications were indeed therapeutic. He eventually abandoned the use of calomel because of its severe side effects.

Although, Jefferson was amenable to his personal use of medicine he was less inclined towards his family's use of it. On two separate occasions he wrote to his daughter Martha respecting the illnesses of two of her children. Concerning a grandson he wrote of how pleased he was that Martha "did not physic him" and, regarding a granddaughter, he cautioned Martha "not to destroy the powers of her stomach with medicine."[22] In all likelihood, Jefferson was addressing the use of mineral (such as calomel) rather than vegetable medicines. In both letters he exhorted Martha not to impede the healing power of nature.

Jefferson's personal acceptance of certain medicines indicates that he viewed them as safer methods of treatment than the unrestrained exertions applied by many physicians. He permitted their use because they induced actions within the body identical to its natural actions. A ". . . fulness [sic] of the stomach we can relieve by emetics; diseases of the bowels, by purgatives; inflammatory cases by bleeding; intermittents, by Peruvian Bark; syphilis, by mercury; watchfulness, by opium; and [etc.] So far, I bow to the utility of medicine."[23] Jefferson explained that past the point of general symptoms and straightforward illnesses the body produced more complicated manifestations of sickness and rather than proceed with unproved medications and haphazard remedies the "judicious, the moral, the humane physician should stop."[24] Jefferson meant that the use of so-called heroic medicine and particular medications were appropriate when brought to bear against ailments known to respond to them; beyond that a doctor's persistent reliance upon them was cruel. He felt that doctors had a predilection for doing just that, however. Quoting Jefferson in his *Personal Memoranda,* Dr. Dunglison wrote "it was not, [Jefferson] was wont to observe, to physic that I object so much as to physicians."[25]

---

22 Harry Bloch, M.D., "Thomas Jefferson 1743 to 1826," *N.Y. State Journal of Medicine* Vol. 72 (1972): p. 3030.

23 John M. Dorsey, M.D., ed., *The Jefferson-Dunglison Letters* (Charlottesville, Virginia: University of Virginia Press, 1960), p. 101.

24 Ibid., p. 102.

As for his own health, Jefferson fell victim to a moderate number of physical ailments during his lifetime. During his early twenties he began to experience severe and debilitating headaches. He suffered with them for most of the remainder of his life. Their cause has never been determined although they were most likely the result of tension. The most effective treatment for him seemed to be lying down and resting in a darkened room, though he did on occasion try Peruvian Bark (quinine) and calomel but experienced no appreciable relief from them.[26] He was tormented by a severe fever in 1783 and again used Peruvian Bark as a treatment.[27] There is no evidence that this was associated with malaria. At some point during his time in France he experienced stomach difficulties. Jefferson purchased pills to treat the condition. The original container, which held the pills, is in the Jefferson collection at Monticello. The small circular box is displayed in the vitrine in Jefferson's bedroom. According to the box's lid the pills are effective against weaknesses of the stomach, constipation and gall bladder complaints. Remember that in 1818 Jefferson experienced a severe case of boils which developed on both buttocks soon after his use of the mineral baths. He was treated for this condition with an ointment containing large amounts of sulphur and mercury. He claimed the treatment almost killed him and he survived only by discontinuing its use.[28]

During the final quarter of his life Jefferson was afflicted with recurring bouts of diarrhea. He described the problem to Benjamin Rush in a letter dated February 28, 1803, believing, he said, that it had originally begun "after having dined moder-

25 Ibid., p. 105.

26 James A. Bear and Gordon Jones, M.D., unpublished monograph of Thomas Jefferson and his health. Monticello Research Archives, 1979.

27 Ibid., p. 7.

28 Ibid., p. 15.

ately on fish which had never affected me before."[29] This affliction was exacerbated several years later, according to Jefferson, by taking the mineral baths in Warm Springs, Virginia. Besides the posterior abscess and boils, Jefferson indicated in his letter that the mineral water had "some small effects on [his] bowels." This suggests that he may have been administered enemas while at the springs.[30]

These "small effects" in time became a major medical problem for Jefferson. They further irritated the bowel condition which he had discussed in his letter to Rush several years earlier. The diarrhea eventually became chronic and necessitated professional visits to Monticello by Dr. Dunglison, who at the time, was serving as professor of medicine at the University of Virginia. The worsening attacks of diarrhea, which Jefferson hid for years from his family, had begun to seriously affect his overall physical state.[31] Jefferson certainly sensed that his deteriorating health was threatening his very life .

About the time Dunglison began his professional calls at Monticello, Jefferson experienced premonitions of mortality. This awareness was exhibited not long before he died. Thomas Jefferson Randolph recalled his grandfather's intuitive feelings of his nearing death which arose during a conversation with him. During that conversation Colonel Randolph was surprised "to hear [Jefferson], in speaking of an event likely to occur about midsummer, say doubtingly that he might live to that time."[32]

In a short time Jefferson's association with the English

---

29 James A. Bear, Jr., Unpublished medical history of Thomas Jefferson, date unknown. p. 643.

30 E. Batts and J. Bear, Jr., eds, *The Family Letters of Thomas Jefferson.* (Columbia, Missouri: University of Missouri Press, 1966), p. 427.

31 Sarah N. Randolph, *The Domestic Life of Thomas Jefferson* (Cambridge, Massachusetts: University Press, 1939), p. 367.

32 Ibid., p. 367.

physician progressed from a professional doctor-patient relationship to a personal friendship of deep mutual admiration. Jefferson had great faith in Dunglison's medical capabilities. On one occasion he told a friend, "I have entire confidence in Dr. Dunglison."[33] A great deal of Jefferson's respect for this gifted physician probably sprang from the fact that Dunglison shared Jefferson's faith in nature's ability to heal and his distaste for extreme treatments.

Dunglison began treating Jefferson during the early months of 1825 and continued until Jefferson's death in July of 1826. Being fully aware of Jefferson's stature and prominence, Dunglison brought all of his considerable skills to bear on Jefferson's case. Jefferson's overriding problems were the continuing attacks of diarrhea and frequent urination. The diarrhea Dunglison treated with laudanum, rhubarb and magnesia. The frequent urination (in all likelihood prostate related) was treated by the insertion of bougie (a long slender device used for dilation) into the urethra.[34] The bougie opened the constriction of the urethra allowing Jefferson's bladder to empty more completely.

What appeared to distress Jefferson as much as the torment of his ailments was the indoor confinement that accompanied them. This constraint was worsened by the fact that he was also bedridden. At the same time, Anne Cary Randolph Bankhead, Jefferson's granddaughter, lay terribly ill and dying at Monticello. In spite of his deep distress over her condition he could not go to her bedside and was unable even to pace the floor in his anxiety. In a letter to her brother, Jefferson wrote, "I have been so ill for several days that I could not go to see her

---

33 Ibid., p. 366.

34 John M. Dorsey, M.D., ed., *The Jefferson-Dunglison Letters* (Charlottesville, Virginia: University of Virginia Press, 1960), p. 38, p. 48.

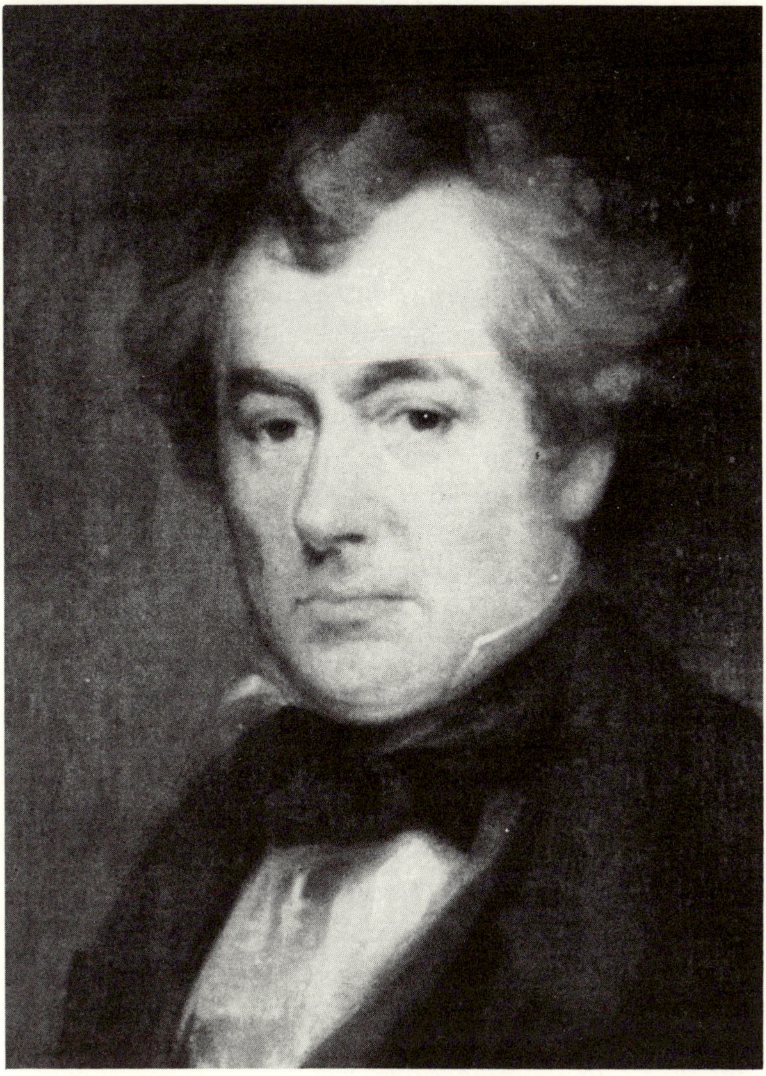

Robley Dunglison

Professor of medicine at the University of Virginia, served as Thomas Jefferson's personal physician. Dunglison eventually convinced the trustees to expand the scope of the School of Medicine. Two years after Jefferson's death, the first Doctor of Medicine degrees were conferred at the University.

Courtesy of Historical Collections and Services, The Claude Moore Health Sciences Library, The University of Virginia

till this morning, and found her speechless and insensible. She breathed her last about 11 o'clock."[35] Jefferson, who had already lost his wife and several of his children, was now deprived of a beloved granddaughter. His anguish must have seemed unbearable. Perhaps, he questioned if living to an elderly age was worth having to watch his beloved family precede him to the grave.

For Jefferson, who was used to spending large amounts of time outdoors, his prostration was certainly frustrating in the extreme. It kept him from his family, his gardens and his riding, the things that seemed best to provide him with relaxation and comfort. His misery can be easily imagined.

Many years before Dr. Dunglison entered the picture, Dr. Rush had recommended to Jefferson some widely prescribed medications to treat his diarrhea. Jefferson mentioned one of these remedies in a letter to William Short, written at Monticello and dated October 31, 1819, "My late illness . . . was produced by a spasmodic stricture of the ileum . . . and I should have been well but that a dose of calomel and jalap, in which were only eight or nine grains of the former, brought on a salivation."[36] Calomel and jalap, both purgatives, were an odd combination with which to treat diarrhea. The blending of the two produced a powerful cathartic (the combination was referred to as Rush's Thunderbolts). In addition, the calomel contained mercury which literally poisoned the user to a degree dependent upon the amount used. Jefferson was quite unhappy that his recovery had been retarded by his use of Rush's remedies.

Dunglison treated Jefferson's diarrhea with gentler medi-

---

35 E. Betts and J. Bear, Jr., eds., *The Family Letters of Thomas Jefferson* (Columbia, Missouri: University of Missouri Press, 1966), p. 470.

36 A. Koch and W. Peden, eds., *The Life and Selected Writings of Thomas Jefferson* (New York: Random House, 1993), p. 633.

cations. Laudanum, a tincture of opium, was prescribed to relax the large intestine and to slow the peristaltic action. The decreased peristaltic action resulted in a reduction of Jefferson's intervals. Dunglison, in a work entitled, *General Therapeutics and Materia Medica,* published in 1843, wrote, "in the inflammations of the lining membrane of the intestinal canal, opium is a most valuable remedy . . . In too great secretion from the mucous membrane of the bowels, it allays, by its sedative agency, the inflammatory or other irritation, and . . . the increased peristaltic action."[37] Dunglison advised Jefferson that should his condition worsen or fail to respond to the prescribed dose then Jefferson should increase the amount taken. Although the use of laudanum did not cure Jefferson, it did enable him to return to the out-of-doors and indulge once again his love of horseback riding, walking and gardening. During November of 1825, Jefferson wrote to Dunglison,

> I certainly cannot say that I am well, but as much so much probably as I ever shall be. I expect to be subject to vacillation of better and worse. My intervals have averaged thro' this month an hour in the day and ¾ in the night with particular instances of 1¾. The day before yesterday I rode about my garden in a walk half an hour without any inconvenience at that time or since, and found it more reviving than in a carriage. I suppose therefore that with care and laudanum I may consider myself in what is to be my habitual state.[38]

Jefferson's prolonged use of opium raises the prospect of opium dependence. Jefferson's reliance on laudanum, with its opium base, and possible earlier uses of other opium-based medicines may well have created an addiction. Jefferson wrote

---

37 John M. Dorsey, M.D., ed., *The Jefferson-Dunglison Letters* (Charlottesville, Virginia: University of Virginia Press, 1960), pp. 50–51.

38 Ibid., pp. 41–42.

to Dunglison that to sustain his "habitual state," or a near normal lifestyle, his use of laudanum would have to be continual. Jefferson had originally been instructed to use twenty-five drops of laudanum per dose to help halt his diarrhea (twenty-five drops of laudanum are approximately equal to one grain of opium). Over time Jefferson's dosage was increased in order to more effectively treat his symptoms. Although opium is less potent than its alkaloids, morphine and codeine, it is still highly addictive. Hence, the increasing dosage of laudanum indicates not only that Jefferson had developed a degree of tolerance to it, requiring greater amounts to control his bowels, but also a possible dependence on the drug.

Several factors would have to be considered before a definitive assessment could be made of an opium dependency. Among these are the number of doses taken per day, the dosage amount and the length of time that Jefferson had been using opium. Individuals differ in their metabolic rate. This influences the amount of opium absorbed into their systems. Depending on his metabolism, Jefferson may have assimilated more or less than some other user. In addition, any deficiency in quality control during the production of laudanum would cause an inconsistency in the strength of each batch produced. This variance would then affect the amount of opium contained in doses from different batches. Despite these qualifiers, which challenge any claim of dependency, the prospect remains intriguing.

A home medical guide, owned by Martha Jefferson Randolph while she was mistress of Monticello, dated April 1824, contains handwritten medicinal recipes that tend to support the probability of routine narcotic usage. Two of the recipes contain opium as an ingredient and would have been useful in treating a bowel condition such as Jefferson's. Their careful placement in the book confirms their use and makes it appear likely that they were prepared to treat Jefferson's troublesome bowel condition. The earlier use of these opiate medications, and the later routine use of laudanum, bolster the possibility of a drug dependence.

Powdered rhubarb and magnesia prescribed by Dunglison in his efforts to arrest Jefferson's diarrhea were, like laudanum, detailed in *General Therapeutics and Materia Medica.* Dunglison explained that though it initially acts as a gentle cathartic, rhubarb later performs as an astringent thus augmenting the effects of the laudanum, and that magnesia, a mild laxative, was prescribed to offset constipation. [39]

Jefferson's warm relationship with Robley Dunglison runs contrary to what might be expected from a man who seemed to possess such little regard for physicians. Possibly it was Dunglison's attitude towards medicine, or his bearing, or his intellect that made him attractive to Jefferson; conceivably, it was all three or none of these. Perhaps, the answer to their close association might lie in Jefferson's authorship of the Declaration of Independence while a slave master. Jefferson was a knotted cord of contradictions. He chastised doctors in general yet sought out their services. He complained of faddish treatments, though he resorted to them himself. And although he used it, he urged that medicine not be given to his grandchildren. All of these inconsistencies proceeded from a man who took the measure of the field of medicine and seemingly concluded *ex nihilo nihil fit,* from nothing comes nothing.

39 Ibid., pp. 49–50.

CHAPTER FOUR

Jefferson and Materia Medica

A Garden Pharmacy

BEFORE THE FINAL DAYS OF WINTER HAD ENDED AT Monticello in 1794, Thomas Jefferson made a series of entries into his *Garden Book*. These entries consisted of a list of the plants he intended to grow that spring. Included was a group he labeled "Objects for the garden this year."[1] Among these objects was an inventory of sixteen herbs. Those herbs and their medicinal properties surely comprised Jefferson's plant pharmacy.

The use of herbs and plants as medicine was widespread in colonial Virginia. For several generations following the founding of the colony, doctors prescribed them and patients self-medicated with them. Needed herbal medications were often filled by an apothecary. Apothecary shops carried large inventories of herbal ingredients and preparations. For instance, a catalog listing the contents of the Williamsburg apothecary shop of Dr. Thomas Wharton contains a sizable number of herbal medicines shipped to him by a London sup-

1 Edwin Morris Betts, ed., *Thomas Jefferson's Garden Book* (Lancaster, Pennsylvania: Lancaster Press, Inc., 1944), p. 212.

plier. Some of the herbal materia medica that Dr. Wharton had on hand were "compound spirits of Lavender, Chamomile Flowers, Salf [sic] of Wormwood, Rhubarb Root, Ointment of Marshmallow, Powdered Sena and Mint."[2] These represent only a small fraction of the herbs and herbal mixtures dispensed by apothecaries in the treatment of illnesses. Many other herbs, such as those grown by Jefferson, were stocked for their therapeutic value.

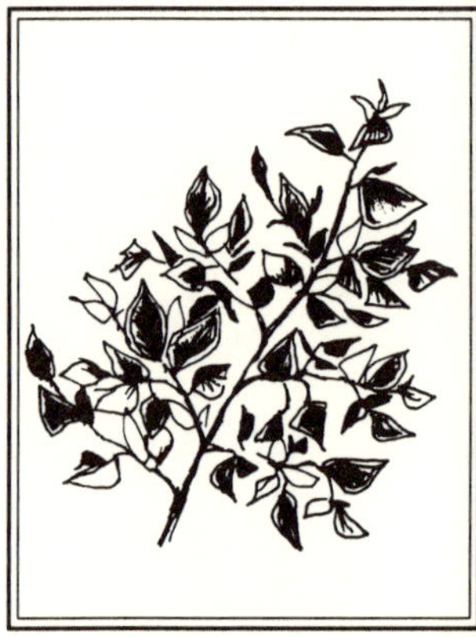

Marjoram
Marjoran hortensis

An illustration of one such herb widely used as medicine and contained among Jefferson's assortment is marjoram. In Nicholas Culpeper's herbal, it says of marjoram, "it is warming and comforting in cold diseases of the head [and] it takes away the inflammation and watering of the eyes."[3] The variety of marjoram grown by Jefferson, *Majorana hortensis,* is a sweet marjoram and would have been quite useful as a kitchen herb, as well. Herbs frequently served dual purposes. The remaining fifteen of Jefferson's herbs were sage, balm, mint, thyme, lavender, chamomile, tansy, rue, wormwood, southernwood, rosemary, hyssop, periwinkle, marshmallow and beargrass.[4] Each herb (beargrass is an exception) has very distinctive medicinal properties and uses. Their virtues were described in the pharmacopoeias and works on physic contained in Jefferson's library. Considering the large number of people living at

---

2 Harold B. Gill, Jr., *The Apothecary in Colonial Virginia* (Williamsburg, Virginia: Colonial Williamsburg Foundation, 1972), pp. 71–75.

3 Nicholas Culpeper, *Culpeper's Complete Herbal* (London: W. Foulsham & Co., Ltd., n.d.), p. 227.

4 Edwin Morris Betts, ed., *Thomas Jefferson's Garden Book: 1766–1824* (Lancaster, Pennsylvania: Lancaster Press, Inc., 1944), p. 208.

Monticello, the need to be familiar with the application of these herbs was important.

Because of their medicinal properties these herbs were highly esteemed. A number of them were considered mainstays in colonial Virginia gardens. Chamomile, lavender, sage, and thyme would have been found in any serious colonial herb patch. They were, however, only as effective as the working knowledge of the user allowed them to be. Jefferson realized this and resolved to be well informed about these botanicals. To this end he acquired a large number of reference volumes such as William Cullen's *A Treatise of the Materia Medica* and *Riverius's Practice of Physic*, by Lazarus Riverius, a volume to which Culpeper had contributed.[5] Other similar works contained in Jefferson's library, and which he undoubtedly read, are listed in E. Millicent Sowerby's *Catalogue of the Library of Thomas Jefferson.* Among them are *Pharmacopoeia Londinensis,* by William Salmon, published in 1682, *Pharmacopoeia Extemporanea,* by Thomas Fuller, published in 1740 and *The Edinburgh New Dispensatory,* by Andrew Duncan, published in 1791.[6] Jefferson's ownership of these herbals, coupled with the cultivation of his many medicinal plants, shows clearly that he intended his herbs to be used for therapeutic purposes.

Certainly, the practice of using herbal and plant medicines to treat illnesses extended well beyond colonial Virginia. Samuel Thomson of New Hampshire, as an example, was a firm believer in the use of herbs as medicines and always treated his family by "administering his favorite emetic herb, lobelia, and infusions of other herbs."[7] In doing so he felt that,

---

5 E. Millicent Sowerby, ed., *Catalogue of the Library of Thomas Jefferson* (Unknown: The Library of Congress, 1952), p. 399, p. 404.

6 Ibid, pp. 397–399.

7 Barbara Griggs, *Green Pharmacy* (Rochester, Vermont: Healing Arts Press, 1991), p. 163.

by employing natural medicaments, he was aiding nature's attempts at healing. Thomson, like Jefferson, believed in *vis medicatrix naturae,* the curative power of nature, and, also like Jefferson, held that it was the doctor's duty to assist, not resist, the natural efforts of the body to heal itself.[8]

In Virginia, as well as in the other dozen colonies, the search was on for botanical remedies. One historian noted the energetic efforts of "Dr. John Mitchell of Urbanna, Virginia, who . . . claimed twenty-five new genera of plants."[9] Many individuals, like Dr. Mitchell, shared the belief that in the vast forests of this new land grew all sorts of plants possessing miraculous cures. It was simply a matter of finding them.

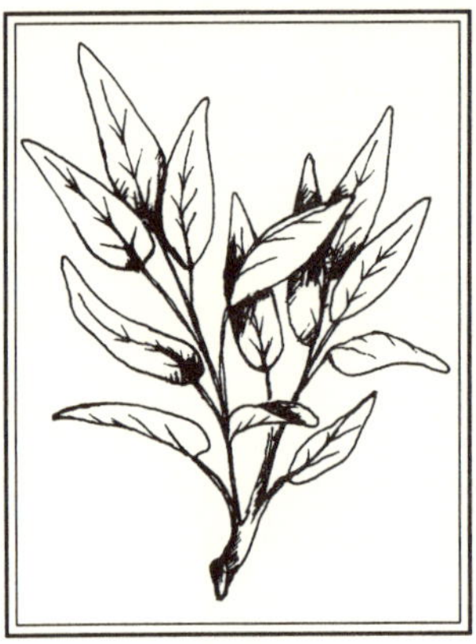

Sage
Salvia officinalis

In the use of vegetable medicines Jefferson was certainly not unique among his equals. Many of his peers either were dosed or dosed themselves with various botanical medications. Two very close associates of Jefferson's, Benjamin Franklin and George Washington, were treated with plant medicines on several occasions. Franklin, who experienced frequent and painful attacks of gout, was purged frequently (no doubt most often with botanic purges) in attempts to alleviate his discomfort.[10] George Washington likewise was purged occasionally and during his final illness, the attending physicians gave him sage tea (an herbal infusion) to use as a gargle to treat his infected throat.[11]

---

8 Ibid., p. 166.

9 Daniel J. Boorstin, *The Americans: The Colonial Experience* (New York: Vintage Books, 1958), p. 213.

10 David Freeman Hawke, *Franklin* (New York: Harper and Row, 1976), p. 280.

11 James Thomas Flexner, *Washington—The Indispensable Man* (Boston: Little, Brown and Company, 1969), p. 399.

Two of the most widely used purges of the time were senna and rhubarb. Rhubarb had been employed in Virginia as a purge since the early 17th century.[12] Both were very effective in their action. Rhubarb played a surprising dual role in that it was also effectual as a treatment for diarrhea.[13] Jefferson cultivated both of these plants at Monticello, as well as lobelia, Samuel Thomson's favorite medicinal plant. *Thomas Jefferson's Garden Book,* edited by Edwin Morris Betts, lists *Rheum undulatum,* an esculent rhubarb, as being planted in April of 1809.[14] Very likely this rhubarb (identified by Betts as *Rheum rhaponticum)* was used medicinally as well as for the table.

Culpeper's Complete Herbal notes that while it is weaker in its purgative properties than other non-esculent rhubarb, *Rheum rhaponticum* is more astringent and thus effective against diarrhea.[15] This characteristic helps explain its selection by Jefferson. Dr. Rush had suggested the use of astringent medicines by Jefferson when he advised him on ways to treat his diarrhea,[16] and Dr. Dunglison, in *General Therapeutics and Materia Medica,* discusses the use of rhubarb as an effective astringent. In fact, rhubarb's ability to bind gave rise to its being referred to as the "constipating purge."[17] During Jefferson's latter days, correspondence between Dunglison and

---

12 Wyndham B. Blanton, *Medicine in Virginia in the Seventeenth Century* (Richmond, Virginia: William Byrd Press, Inc., 1930), p. 12.

13 Barbara Griggs, *Green Pharmacy* (Rochester, Vermont: Healing Arts Press, 1991), pp. 27–28.

14 Edwin Morris Betts, ed., *Thomas Jefferson's Garden Book* (Lancaster, Pennsylvania: Lancaster Press, Inc., 1944), p. 385.

15 Nicholas Culpeper, *Culpeper's Complete Herbal* (London: W. Foulsham & Co., Ltd., n.d.), p. 292.

16 James A. Bear, Jr., Unpublished Medical Chronology of Thomas Jefferson. Monticello Research Archives, n.d., p. 645.

17 Norman Taylor, *Plant Drugs that Changed the World* (New York: Dodd, Mead & Company, 1965), p. 157.

Jefferson notes the treatment of Jefferson's spastic bowels with rhubarb.[18] The astringent property of *Rheum rhaponticum* was exactly what Jefferson needed to deal with his recurring bouts of diarrhea. In all probability, Jefferson, prior to Dunglison's arrival, had consulted his pharmacopoeias and learned that this variety of rhubarb was a specific for treating his condition. Again, it seems quite probable that Jefferson grew this particular variety of rhubarb for its curative, as well as table value.

Senna appears in Jefferson's *Garden Book* as early as 1786. In a letter to his farm manager dated December 19th of that year, Jefferson wrote that he had forwarded bladder senna to Monticello to be planted.[19] Culpeper explains that senna and rhubarb are very similar in their respective purging actions.[20] The 1786 planting of senna precedes the onset of Jefferson's chronic diarrhea by fifteen years. Clearly, senna was grown for use as a laxative.

Botanical purges were considered an integral part of therapy employed against diseases.[21] Monticello's large population certainly found frequent need for the medicinal application of these two plants. Today, laxatives containing senna are still employed to relieve simple constipation.

Another non-herb plant, medicinally useful, which Jefferson grew was the benne (*Sesamum trifoliatum*) or sesame plant. He especially enjoyed the oil extracted from the benne seed. Jefferson claimed, in a letter to John Taylor, that when eaten on a salad it was found to be "equal to the olive oil."[22] In

---

18 John M. Dorsey, M.D., *The Jefferson-Dunglison Letters* (Charlottesville, Virginia: University of Virginia Press, 1960), p. 48.

19 Edwin Morris Betts, ed., *Thomas Jefferson's Garden Book* (Lancaster, Pennsylvania: Lancaster Press, Inc., 1944), p. 118.

20 Nicholas Culpeper, *Culpeper's Complete Herbal* (London: W. Foulsham & Co., Ltd., n.d.), p. 329.

21 Harold B. Gill, Jr., *The Apothecary in Colonial Virginia* (Williamsburg, Virginia: Colonial Williamsburg Foundation, 1972), p. 47.

a later letter Jefferson cited the benne plant's usefulness as a medicine. To Dr. Gustavus Horner, Jefferson explained that "the leaf is a specific in dysenteries & other visceral complaints. Two or three without being bruised, being put into a pint of cold water, in a few minutes produce a mucilage equal to that of the white of an egg. 5. or 6. pints are taken in the course of the day."[23] Jefferson's informed description of the benne plant's effectiveness against intestinal disorders and the fact that he suffered from such a disorder is surely not coincidental. Jefferson apparently used the remedy himself.

Jefferson's knowledge of botanical medicine is an example of the vast range of intellectual curiosity he possessed. He was fascinated by all aspects of nature and, as evidenced by his faith in natural healing, eagerly sought out the harmonic relationship between man and his environment. His respect for nature undoubtedly was responsible for his belief that botany was one of the most valuable of all the sciences.[24] He explained his reasoning for this, in a letter to Thomas Cooper in 1814 in which he listed the numerous ways that plants serve man. One of the principal ways, Jefferson wrote, is "as furnishing . . . medicaments for our bodies."[25] Jefferson undertook such extensive work in the science of botany that a plant was named in his honor, *Jeffersonia diphylla* (a flowering herbaceous plant), in recognition of the significant contributions which he had made to natural history.[26]

Jefferson was certainly intrigued by the therapeutic value

---

22 Edwin Morris Betts, ed., *Thomas Jefferson's Garden Book* (Lancaster, Pennsylvania: Lancaster Press, Inc., 1944), p. 362.

23 Ibid., p. 371.

24 E. Millicent Sowerby, *Catalogue of the Library of Thomas Jefferson* (unknown: The Library of Congress, 1952), p. 479.

25 Ibid.

26 Dumas Malone, *Jefferson and the Rights of Man* (Boston: Little, Brown and Company, 1951), p. 446.

of the herbs and several other plants grown at Monticello. His interest, however, was not confined just to the plants that he grew. One that he did not grow seems to have particularly aroused his interest as an alternative for patients suffering from incurable diseases. In a letter to Dr. Samuel Brown dated July 14, 1813, Jefferson addressed the use of the plant *Datura-Stramomium* or James-Town weed. He suggested to Dr. Brown that a lethal drug produced from the plant, if "restrained to self-administration," be made available to individuals wishing to relieve themselves from the afflictions of terminal illness.[27] The plant, wrote Jefferson, brings on death as gently as "fatigue does ordinary sleep."[28] That Jefferson would make this proposition to a man dedicated to preserving life clearly indicates how strongly he felt about the issue and how comfortable he was with the societal implications of the process.

Like many of Jefferson's ideas, this one was ahead of its time. American society is only now beginning to seriously debate the moral and ethical dilemma of doctor-assisted death. Activist Dr. Jack Kevorkian, himself involved in numerous physician-assisted suicides, has forcibly placed this issue before the court of public opinion. Jefferson was at ease with the moral and ethical concerns associated with such action and overtly promoted its implementation almost two hundred years before Dr. Kevorkian's advocacy.

Jefferson's endorsement for the use of James-Town weed highlights two significant points. First, if a plant or herb held the power to alleviate suffering, Jefferson advocated its use. Second, it is a short step from advocacy to action. Therefore,

---

27 A. Koch and W. Peden, eds., *The Life and Selected Writings of Thomas Jefferson* (New York: Random House, 1993), pp. 575–576.
28 Ibid.

mindful of the therapeutic value of the various herbs and plants at Monticello, Jefferson would have readily used them to treat himself and his family.

In 1813 the same Dr. Brown sent Jefferson a package of Capsicum (pepper plants).[29] Capsicum's popularity as a medication sprang from its effectiveness as a gastric and intestinal stimulant and as a means of treating aches within the joints.[30] Jefferson experienced the first of many episodes of joint pain in about 1794. This condition tormented him, periodically, for most of the remainder of his life. He mentioned one of these painful incidences in a letter to Martha, written from Washington, November 1, 1808. Jefferson wrote her, "as soon as my atack [sic] of rheumatism came on, I applied flannel to the part and toasted a great deal before the fire. It carried it off completely in four days . . . ."[31] Jefferson was obviously familiar with the benefits of exposing the affected area to heat. The successful treatment described to Martha was apparently one he had used before.

A topical medication to "heat" the distressed joint would have been a distinct and welcomed improvement over the flannel and fire. Should an attack have occurred during warm weather the heavy wrapping and intense heat from a fire would have been torturous. Dr. Brown's Capsicum was for Jefferson "just what the doctor ordered."

Pepper had for some time been "considered a heating drug."[32] Culpeper declared it effective when applied as a poul-

---

29 Edwin Morris Betts, ed., *Thomas Jefferson's Garden Book: 1766–1824* (Lancaster, Pennsylvania: Lancaster Press, Inc., 1944), p. 514.

30 Barbara Griggs, *Green Pharmacy* (Rochester, Vermont: Healing Arts Press, 1991), pp.166–167.

31 E. Betts and J. Bear, Jr., eds., *The Family Letters of Thomas Jefferson* (Columbia, Missouri: University of Missouri Press, 1966), p. 355.

32 Harold B. Gill, Jr., *The Apothecary in Colonial Virginia* (Williamsburg, Virginia: Colonial Williamsburg Foundation, 1972), p. 2.

tice against inflammation and pain.[33] That Dr. Robert Brown of Richmond, Virginia was a proponent of its use was evidenced by an inventory of his estate which listed the sizable amount of "1¾ lb Pepper."[34] In a letter dated August 26, 1811, Rush wrote to Jefferson prescribing "bathing [Jefferson's rheumatic] parts with a liniment . . . in which a tablespoon of cayenne pepper has been mixed. . . . "[35]

Jefferson had been growing pepper grass and could now add the Capsicum to his medicinal inventory. He wrote to Dr. Brown expressing appreciation for the supply of the plant sent by him adding that he would "set great store by the Capsicum. . . ."[36] Jefferson's expressed appreciation for the Capsicum was owing in part to a progressive worsening of his rheumatism. Two years earlier he had written Dr. Rush, "I have had a long attack of rheumatism . . . A total prostration of the muscles of the back, hips and thighs, deprived me of the power of walking, and leaves it still in a very impaired state. A pain when I walk seems to have fixed itself in the hip, and seems to threaten permanence. . . ."[37] There was an additional benefit in the Capsicum for Jefferson's ailing muscles; *Culpeper's Complete Herbal* recommends it for use against the discomfort of a troublesome back.[38]

---

33 Nicholas Culpeper, *Culpeper's Complete Herbal* (London: W. Foulsham & Co., Ltd.,n.d.), p. 270

34 Harold B. Gill, Jr., *The Apothecary in Colonial Virginia* (Williamsburg, Virginia: Colonial Williamsburg Foundation, 1972), p. 77.

35 Mary Marquis, *A Short Synopsis of the Uses of Medicinal Plants-Herbs-from Past to Present.* Unpublished paper presented to the University of Virginia, February 10, 1995.

36 Edwin Morris Betts, ed., *Thomas Jefferson's Garden Book* (Lancaster, Pennsylvania: Lancaster Press, Inc., 1944), p. 517.

37 J.A. Bear, Jr. and G. Jones, M.D., *Thomas Jefferson and His Health* (None: Unpublished, None), p. 13.

38 Nicholas Culpeper, *Culpeper's Complete Herbal* (London: W. Foulsham & Co., Ltd., n.d.), p. 270.

The remaining herbs grown in Jefferson's garden offered medicinal benefits that could be employed to treat any number of illnesses. Rue, tansy, southernwood, wormwood, hyssop, balm and rosemary all contributed to help heal the sick and restore health to the household. The effective use of these herbs simply required familiarity with their capabilities. Owning medical books was a great help. As befits a practical man, in this regard, Jefferson was well prepared.

Thomas Jefferson was not a person to own a book and not read it. Reading was one of his passions. This was evidenced by the breadth of his library. His vast knowledge had not come solely from observation and experience. To Charles Bellini, professor of modern languages at the College of William and Mary, Jefferson wrote, "books, really good, . . . communicate to us all their advances in knowledge."[39] One of his granddaughters recalled Jefferson's devotion to books and reading. "He studied fifteen hours a day. During the most closely occupied days of his college life it was his habit to study until two o'clock at night . . . during vacations . . . he still devoted nearly three-fourths of his time to his books."[40] Jefferson retained this passion for reading throughout his life. Writing to his friend, Rush, late in life, Jefferson proclaimed, "I have fixed myself comfortably, keep some books here [Poplar Forest], bring others occasionally. . . ."[41]

Evidence that Jefferson read his medical volumes in depth is the long-term correspondence he maintained with several physicians. Many of these doctors were recognized in

39 A. Koch and W. Peden, eds., *The Life and Selected Writings of Thomas Jefferson* (New York: Random House, 1993), p. 355.

40 Sarah N. Randolph, *The Domestic Life of Thomas Jefferson* (Cambridge, Massachusetts: University Press, 1939), p. 15.

41 A. Koch and W. Peden, eds., *The Life and Selected Writings of Thomas Jefferson* (New York: Random House, 1993), p. 562.

their time as among the most powerful men in the field of medicine. Rush, for instance, and his theories influenced the American medical field for decades. Dunglison was a force in his profession and possessed, throughout his lifetime, an excellent reputation within the medical community. Other notable doctors with whom Jefferson corresponded were George Gilmer Jr., Gustavus Horner and Samuel Brown, all highly regarded. Gilmer, a neighbor and close friend, attended Jefferson and his family at Monticello for many years. Men of such eminent standing would not have fashioned an association with Jefferson if they had not respected his knowledge and understanding of their profession. Such familiarity could only have come from extensive reading of his medical volumes. Jefferson may have lacked the skills to practice medicine but he had a firm grasp on the details.

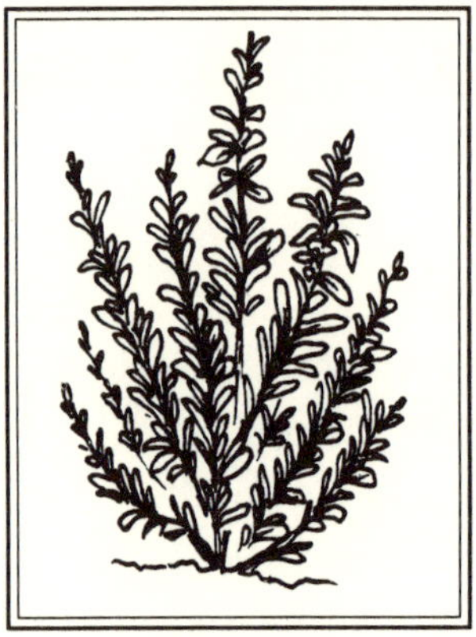

Rosemary
Rosemarinus officinalis

As a consequence of his readings, Jefferson was familiar with the therapeutic uses of herbs and plants. The specifics of the materia medica were known to him. If, however, he found it necessary, his books were always available for quick reference. Dr. John M. Dorsey points out that Jefferson's personal copy of Robert Thomas' *Modern Practice of Physic* was well worn and "opened easiest to its section dealing with intestinal disorders."[42] With Jefferson's history of episodic diarrhea, it takes little imagination to picture him thumbing through the pages searching for remedies.

Several herbals contained in Jefferson's library have been previously mentioned. Detailing the therapeutic usage of a vast

42 John M. Dorsey, M.D., ed., *The Jefferson-Dunglison Letters* (Charlottesville, Virginia: University of Virginia Press, 1960), p. 96.

array of herbs and plants, they provided Jefferson with an abundance of information. These herbals were some of the most popular of their time. They provided readers with straightforward advice on the preparation and use of botanical medications. Using simple language and instructions these books guided laymen through the process of reducing herbs and plants to useful medicines. Most of the preparations described were simple teas, powders, poultices and the like. Yet, for the people who used them, great faith was placed in their effectiveness. Compared with today's sophisticated medicines most of these early remedies had little more curative value than sugar pills.

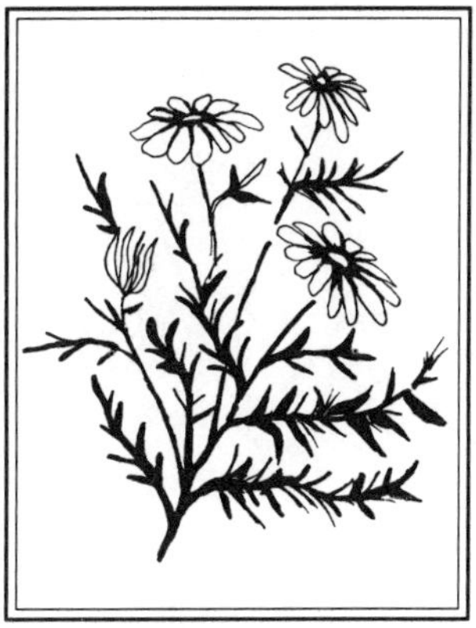

Chamomile
Anthemis nobilis

The level of Jefferson's interest in self-prepared botanical medicines was heightened by the fact that no doctor was involved in the treatment. Jefferson most certainly viewed self-treatment as a safer method of healthcare. Any physician reckless enough to advocate bleeding over chamomile tea for indigestion would have met with disdain from Jefferson. Drinking a cup of soothing herbal tea was sensible, it had been proven effective. Bleeding, was at best, of dubious value and at worst a total sham.

Some of Monticello's herbs, surely to Jefferson's delight, were suitable for dual use; they could season food as well as dose the sick. Sage, thyme, marjoram, mint and rosemary were apropos for food preparation, as well as medicine. Others such as rue, wormwood, southernwood, and tansy were strictly medicinal herbs. Regardless of their respective categories, all of Jefferson's herbs represented a frail, yet trusted, wall of protection against the effects of disease for him and his family.

Along with occasional visits from the doctor they were the only response available to illness.

Sage (*Salvia officinalis*), derived from a word meaning healthy, had been highly regarded since antiquity. Sage, according to Culpeper, "stays the bleeding of wounds and cleanses foul ulcers or sores."[43] Cullen, in his *Materia Medica,* asserts that sage contains a volatile oil that can be used as a sudorific (sweat inducer) with the patient wrapped tightly from head to foot and is effective also in the prevention of violent spasms caused by intermittent fevers, common in colonial Virginia.[44] Balm (*Melissa officinalis*), an aromatic plant and a medicinal complement to sage, was used to prepare a tea alleged to control all types of fevers.[45] Over time, sage became primarily a culinary herb; balm, however, is still used by herbalists and homeopathic practitioners to treat fevers.[46]

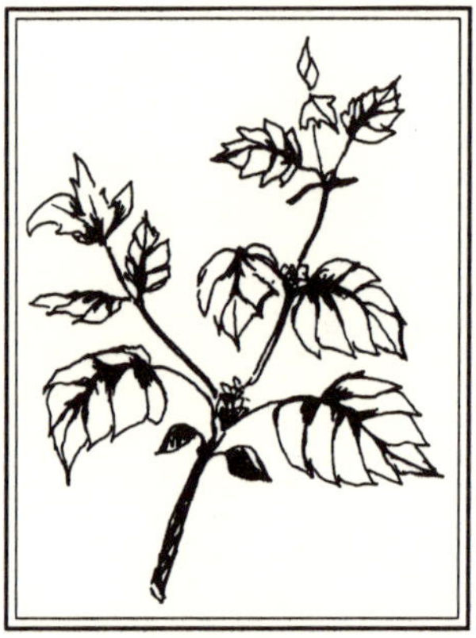

Balm
Melissa officinalis

Fevers were cause for great concern in Jefferson's day, for frequently they signaled the onslaught of a serious disease. One such disease characterized by periodic fever (an ague) and marked by regularly recurring chills is, today, known worldwide as malaria.[47] In tandem with Peruvian Bark, Jefferson

43 Nicholas Culpeper, *Culpeper's Complete Herbal* (London: W. Foulsham & Co., Ltd., n.d.), p. 311.

44 William Cullen, *A Treatise of the Materia Medica* (Edinburgh, Scotland: Unknown, 1789), p. 103.

45 Ibid., p. 466.

46 J. Dwyer and D. Rattray, eds., *Magic and Medicine of Plants* (Pleasantville, New York: Reader's Digest Association, Inc., 1993), p. 90.

47 Norman Taylor, *Plant Drugs that Changed the World* (New York: Dodd, Mead & Company, 1965), p. 74.

could easily have resorted to the use of sage and balm to help reduce the severity of these dreaded fevers when they struck.[48]

Mint (*Mentha piperita*), one of the more prevalent garden herbs, originated in the Near East and was one of the first cultivated herbs to travel to the colonies.[49] Described by Cullen as being effective as a digestive aid and against gripping, the pinching, spasmodic pain associated with diarrhea, this herb would have been ideal for use by Jefferson to ease his cramping.[50] On one occasion in 1803, Jefferson wrote Benjamin Rush complaining of his protracted diarrhea and that his "bowels . . . are weak and labor in their operations . . . ."[51] Rush replied, telling Jefferson that "peppermint tea may be taken occasionally . . . for paroxysms of your disease."[52] Peppermint tea was a simple prescription and apparently proved effective for Jefferson grew a ready supply of the active ingredient in his garden.

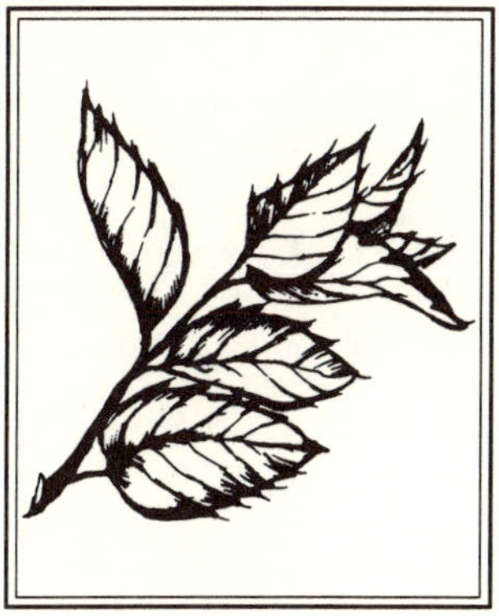

Mint
Mentha piperita

As an adult, Jefferson experienced a few episodes of aching teeth. In a letter to Martha, he wrote, "I was taken with a tooth-ache about 5. days ago, which brought on a very large and hard swelling of the face, and that produced a fever . . ." and, shortly thereafter wrote to his granddaughter, Ellen Wayles Randolph, "my swelled face is not yet entirely well."[53] Jefferson

48 Ibid., p. 79.

49 M. Marquis and L. Richmond, *Objects for the Garden: Useful Plants from Jefferson's Time* (Unknown: Unknown, 1994), p. 11.

50 William Cullen, *A Treatise of the Materia Medica* (Edinburgh, Scotland: Unknown, 1789), p. 540.

51 James A. Bear, Jr., *Unpublished medical chronology of Thomas Jefferson.* Monticello Research Archives, n.d., p. 643.

52 Ibid.

53 E. Betts and J. Bear, Jr., eds., *The Family Letters of Thomas Jefferson* (Columbia, Missouri: University of Missouri Press, 1966), p. 317, p. 330.

continued to experience problems with his teeth for some time afterwards as described in letters written more than a year later, again to Martha and Ellen, in which he complained of his "diseased jaw."[54] Thyme (*Thymus vulgaris*) was listed in Jefferson's copy of *The Edinburgh New Dispensatory* as containing an oil with which a sufferer might seek relief from tooth pain.[55] It is likely that Jefferson's aching teeth and later tooth afflictions prompted him to seek the pain-relieving properties of this herb. Beyond its recommended use for tooth pain Jefferson may have employed thyme to help against his bowel misery. Culpeper noted that "it purges the body of phlegm [and] comforts the stomach much and expels wind."[56]

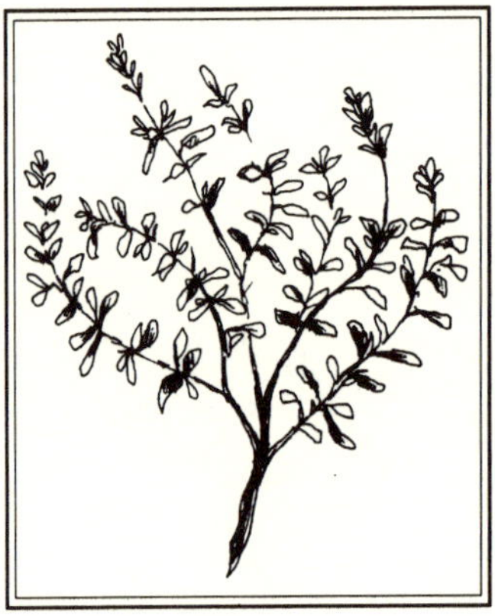

Thyme
Thymus vulgaris

Lavender (*Lavandula spica*), immensely popular in England, became equally as popular in colonial gardens.[57] Its slender spiked stems and purplish-blue flowers could have been easily spotted among the other garden herbs. While appreciated for its strong but pleasant fragrance, and as a house freshener, it was also heralded by the herbals of Jefferson's day as a valuable medicine. According to the *Edinburgh New Dispensatory*, lavender converted into a tincture, oil or spirit was good for "vertigoes, palsies, tremors, disorders of the head,

54 Ibid., p. 330.

55 Andrew Duncan, *The Edinburgh New Dispensatory* (Philadelphia: T. Dobson, 1791), p. 297.

56 Nicholas Culpeper, *Culpeper's Complete Herbal* (London: W. Foulsham & Co., Ltd., n.d.), p. 371.

57 Colonial Dames of America, *Herbs and Herb Lore of Colonial America* (New York: Dover Publications, Inc., 1995), p. 33.

nerves and uterus."[58] Culpeper's herbal prescribes it as "of especial use in pains of the head and brain . . . ."[59] This quality could have held great appeal for Jefferson.

For many years, Jefferson experienced what he referred to as "periodical headaches." The headaches were generally of several weeks duration and generated intense pain, especially at the onset.[60] Jefferson mentioned his unpleasant experiences with these headaches in letters to friends and family throughout his life. To Martha he wrote in May 1790, "I hoped to have been soon rid of the periodical headache which had attacked me."[61] Jefferson, suffering sharp pain, closed the letter quickly telling Martha that his head prevented him from writing at length. In 1807, again in a letter to Martha, he informed her that "I am now in the 7th day of a periodical head-ache . . . The fits . . . hold me very long, from 9. or 10. in the morning till dark. Neither Calomel nor bark have as yet made the least impression on them."[62] In the absence of any relief from the medications he described, Jefferson would certainly have sought out other remedies to alleviate his suffering. Since lavender was recommended by Jefferson's herbals for afflictions of the head, his severe headaches and cultivation of lavender suggest that he may well have used the herb to treat his symptoms. Inasmuch as Jefferson was

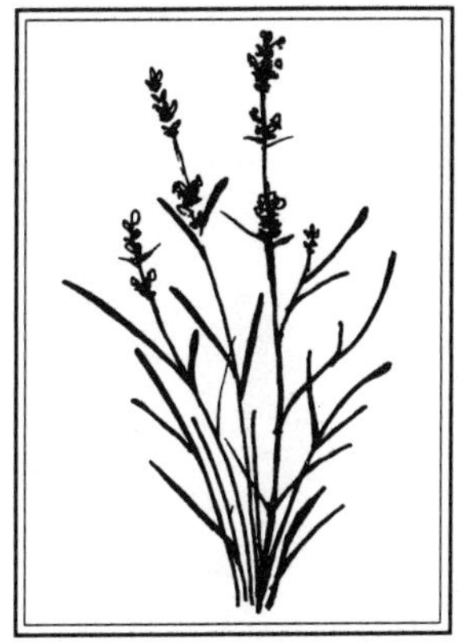

Lavender
Lavendula spica

58 Andrew Duncan, *The Edinburgh New Dispensatory* (Philadelphia: T. Dobson, 1791), p. 218.

59 Nicholas Culpeper, *Culpeper's Complete Herbal* (London: W. Foulsham & Co., Ltd., n.d.), p. 210.

60 J.A. Bear, Jr. and G. Jones, M.D., *Thomas Jefferson and His Health* (None: Unpublished, None), p. 13.

61 E. Betts and J. Bear, Jr., eds., *The Family Letters of Thomas Jefferson* (Columbia, Missouri: University of Missouri Press, 1966), p. 56.

62 Ibid., p. 304.

agreeable to trying calomel (a purgative) and Peruvian Bark as the means to control his headaches, there is no reason to doubt that he might have tried the lavender medication as well.

Chamomile (*Anthemis nobilis*) and tansy (*Tanacetum vulgare*) are both cited in numerous Jefferson-owned herbals. Chamomile, steeped in hot water, produced a beneficial tea. According to Cullen's, *A Treatise of the Materia Medica,* chamomile tea was "excellent to warm and strengthen the stomach, in cases of indigestion, loss of appetite, and other complaints arising from debility."[63] Many people today find chamomile tea useful against indigestion and as a soothing drink before retiring at night. Tansy, according to William Salmon's *Pharmacopeia Londinensis,* was excellent for cleansing "the stomach and bowels of harmful matter."[64] Given their medicinal qualities, it can be assumed that Jefferson used these two herbs to treat his bowel infirmity and other digestive complaints.

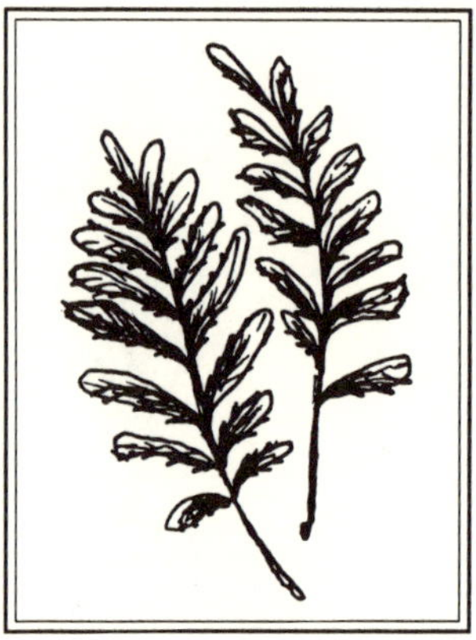

Tansy
Tanacetum vulgare

Rue (*Ruta graveolens*), another Monticello herb, was recommended, when applied topically, for the stings of bees and wasps and when taken internally as an aid against cramps and colic.[65] Not only Jefferson, but also his grandchildren, might well have had need of this herb. From early spring till mid-fall, Monticello boasted a wide variety of blooming flowers. As a consequence, there would have been an abundance of bees capable at any moment of delivering a painful sting. And, a

63 William Cullen, *A Treatise of the Materia Medica* (Edinburgh, Scotland: Unknown, 1789), p. 477.

64 William Salmon, *Pharmacopoeia Londinensis* (London: Unknown, 1682), p. 107.

65 Ibid., p. 59.

grandchild suffering a late night attack of colic could have kept the household awake until a dose of rue restored the child's slumber. In both cases the parents', not to mention grandfather Jefferson's, appreciation for rue's capabilities can be easily imagined. As for Jefferson personally, his probable use of rue as an aid against cramping is by now clear.

Rue also served as an anthelmintic. Anthelmintics were used to destroy intestinal worms. It is easy to imagine the children, black and white, living at Monticello, placing dirty hands in their mouths or running outside barefoot, contracting internal parasites. For children as well as adults of the time, intestinal parasites were common.[66] A good dosing with rue would have been in order.

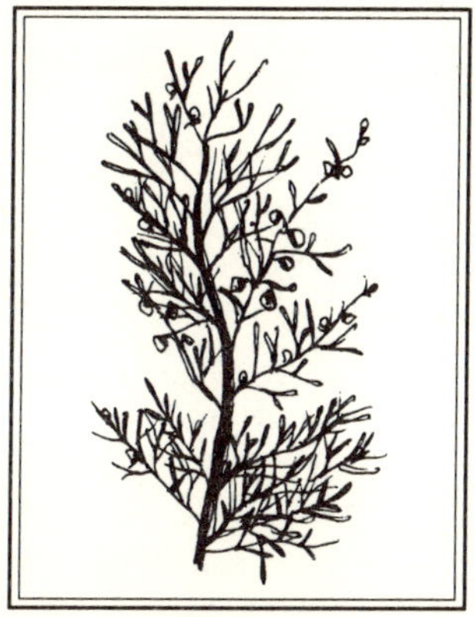

Wormwood
Artemisia absinthum

Wormwood (*Artemisia absinthium*) and southernwood (*Artemisia abrotanum*) further supplied Jefferson with botanic medicaments. Like rue, southernwood was highly regarded as a treatment for intestinal worms and also as a purgative.[67] Wormwood was suggested for use "to strengthen the stomach [and] digestion . . . It is good in all agues."[68] Jefferson may have formed a special attachment to this, along with the other herbs that were identified as specific in ailments of the alimentary canal. Patented stomach pills, such as those he had procured in France, were costly. Herbal treatments were free and, in all likelihood, just as effective.

66 J. Dwyer and D. Rattray, eds., *Magic and Medicine of Plants* (Pleasantville, New York: Reader's Digest Association, Inc., 1993), p. 286.

67 William Cullen, *A Treatise of the Materia Medica* (Edinburgh, Scotland: Unknown, 1789), p. 55.

68 Nicholas Culpeper, *Culpeper's Complete Herbal* (London: W. Foulsham & Co., Ltd., n.d.), pp. 394–396.

Salmon's *Pharmacopoeia Londinensis* identifies the benefits of four of the remaining five herbs. They are rosemary (*Rosmarinus officinalis*), hyssop (*Hyssopus officinalis*), periwinkle (variety unknown, likely *Vinca minor*) and marshmallow (*Althaea officinalis*). Salmon states that rosemary is effective as a cephalic, a medication used to treat problems of the head. Hyssop is specific as a purge and useful against lung problems and tumors. Periwinkle is described as effective against toothaches and to control bleeding. Marshmallow was also urged for use in dealing with acrimony (ill-temper), pleurisies and pains in the side.[69] Culpeper, in his herbal, further explains that marshmallow can be used to produce a "mucilage of the roots . . . much used in poultices [for inflammation]."[70] Many of the aforementioned ailments treated by these herbs Jefferson had either experienced personally or realized could strike someone at Monticello at anytime. Several among them: headache, toothache, bleeding, inflammations and muscle aches, were common occurrences. The large number of people living, playing and working at Monticello guaranteed that almost everyday someone would suffer one or another such affliction requiring the use of medicinal herbs. Jefferson no doubt foresaw these eventualities when preparing his list of herbs to be planted.

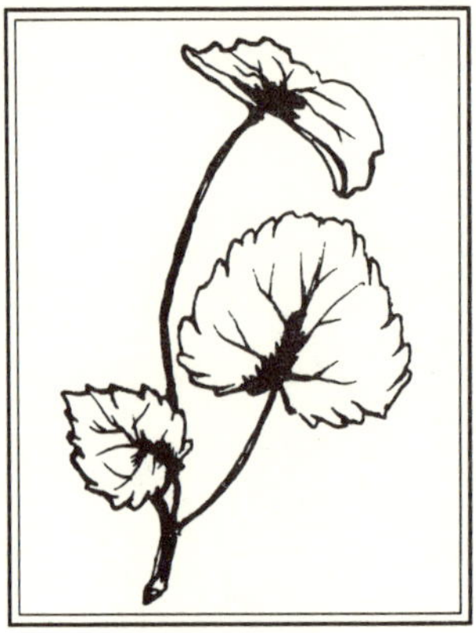

Marshmallow
Althaea officinalis

The last herb listed by Jefferson in the 1794 herb group is beargrass (*Yucca filamentosa*). Beargrass, a member of the lily family, is a tough fibrous plant possessing grasslike leaves and

---

69 William Salmon, *Pharmacopoeia Londinensis* (London: Unknown, 1682), pp. 25–65.

70 Nicholas Culpeper, *Culpeper's Complete Herbal* (London: W. Foulsham & Co., Ltd., n.d.), p. 225.

producing diminutive white flowers. Its use by Jefferson is unclear. The little bit that is known includes the fact that the white flowers are edible and can be used in dishes such as salads. The possibility that Jefferson might have used the plant for food is conjecture. Jefferson's *Garden Book* suggests that the filament-like leaves may have been used to tie up bundles of plant items for storage.

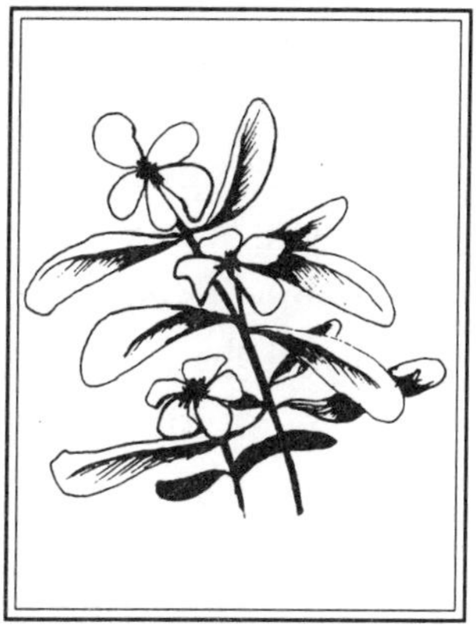

Periwinkle
Vinca minor

Why did Jefferson leave no known record of how he used his herbs? Perhaps because during his lifetime the woman of the house "doctored" the family. As Catherine Clinton has pointed out, "the female head of the household acted as doctor or nurse . . . for it was her task to supervise the medical care of her families, white and black. She oversaw the daily dispensation of the medicine . . . [and] physicians called only when the white family's needs had exhausted the plantation mistress's curative powers."[71] After the death of his wife Martha, and owing to Jefferson's subsequent unwillingness to remarry, Martha Jefferson Randolph, Jefferson's eldest daughter and wife of Thomas Mann Randolph, in time became mistress of Monticello. Her responsibilities, which she accepted gladly, included the care of her father. On March 20, 1807, she wrote to Jefferson, "I make no exception when I say the first and most important object with me will be the dear and sacred duty of nursing and chearing [sic] your old age by every endearment of filial tenderness."[72] Clearly, Martha was prepared to devote herself to making her

---

71 Catherine Clinton, *The Plantation Mistress* (New York: Pantheon Books, 1982), p. 143.

72 Dumas Malone, *Jefferson the President,* vol. 5, *Jefferson And His Time* (Boston: Little, Brown and Company, 1974), p. 144.

father happy and dedicated to guarding his health during his final years. This "in-house" health care was a general household affair. It would not have warranted meticulous record keeping.

The only room in the house suitable for the preparation of medicines and possessing all of the implements necessary was the kitchen. Appropriately, the ingredients and the instructions for compounding them were generally written as recipes. Then, as now, women held dominion over this area of the home. As mistress of Monticello, Martha would have supervised the kitchen and had the responsibility of preparing, as well as administering, medications. This arrangement is supported by a recent find at Monticello. During renovations at the home, boxed artifacts were located dating back to the time of Martha's residence. One of these was a medical book entitled *Modern Practice of Physic,* written by Robert Thomas, MD. Its physical appearance bears witness to frequent use, indicating that this 1822 publication was heavily relied on by the family. A notation at the top of the title page reads, "Govr. [Thomas Mann] Randolph from his friend D. Hosack" and inside the front cover is written "M[artha] Randolph Monticello April 26, 1824." Thomas Mann Randolph evidently accepted the small gift and then turned it over to his wife, Martha. The fact that the book was given over to Martha clearly corroborates her role as the family's primary health care provider. The final flyleaf and inside back cover contain several handwritten recipes for remedies and cures. There are, in addition, many newspaper clippings dealing with medicinal treatments pasted onto the front and back endpapers. Martha's health care responsibilities, along with her ownership of this volume, which preceded Jefferson's death by more than two years, lends substantial weight to the likelihood that Jefferson was administered at least some of the treatments contained therein.

Two of the handwritten medicinal recipes are of particular interest as both contain opium. The drug, often referred to as "God's own medicine," helped check Jefferson's chronic diarrhea. Opium, as reviewed earlier, played a significant role in Jefferson's health care near the end of his life and perhaps sooner. The two recipes in question, "camphor and opium pills" and "rye water," may have been used to treat Jefferson prior to Dr. Dunglison's arrival in early 1825. The camphor and opium pill recipe (per dose) called for 1½ grains of opium, or 40 drops of laudanum, with 4 grains of camphor (camphor and opium are the primary ingredients of a later tincture called paregoric). Camphor, a tough, gummy substance obtained from the camphor tree, works medicinally as a carminative to expel gas from the alimentary canal. Its texture allowed the resulting compound to be rolled into pill form. Jefferson had been aware for some time of opium's beneficial effect on diarrhea. In the letter, noted earlier, from Rush to Jefferson in 1803 responding to Jefferson's complaint of diarrhea, Rush recommended the use of opium to control the intervals and any pain that might accompany them. Rush wrote that forty drops of laudanum mixed in water would ease Jefferson's discomfort.[73] The identical amounts of laudanum recommended in Rush's letter and the recipe are intriguing and presumably not coincidental, especially as the recipe is handwritten and not a part of the text of Thomas's book. In keeping with Jefferson's penchant for details, he may well have jotted down this formula years earlier for safekeeping.

The rye water recipe calls for a teaspoon of laudanum, water and white vitriol (to prevent constipation) which likewise is extremely similar to Rush's advice to Jefferson to use lauda-

73 James A. Bear, Jr., *Unpublished medical chronology of Thomas Jefferson.* Monticello Research Archives, n.d., p. 645.

num mixed in water to control Jefferson's intervals and uneasiness (in other words calm his nerves). Both medicinal recipes were specific for the treatment of alimentary canal and lower bowel problems identical to those suffered by Jefferson and could very well have been used by him for that purpose.

From Jefferson's memorandum books it is possible to determine some of the medications that he purchased for use at home. Spanning the years 1767 to 1826, the books have recently been edited by James A. Bear, Jr. and Lucia C. Stanton. They provide an interesting and detailed account of Jefferson's business transactions. Maintaining these accounts allowed Jefferson to keep a running list of expenditures not only for medicine but also for other consumable items such as his large wine reserve. Being meticulous, Jefferson believed that he might, by this method, track excessive or frivolous use. For instance an entry for April 7, 1775, notes that "In three months and one week . . . we have used at Elk Hill [one of Jefferson's farms] 2. doz. bottles of Madeira, 3 bottles of red wine, & 10. pint flasks of Syracuse which is at the rate of 10. bottles a month."[74] An example of how exact Jefferson was is an entry dated May 17, 1784, "Pd. for 2 tickets to see balon on 15/."[75] The purchase of two tickets to view a hot air balloon was, after all, an expenditure and as such required recording.

Jefferson evidently made frequent use of Peruvian Bark (also called Jesuits bark or bark) perhaps for his "periodical headaches" but definitely to treat fevers. Scattered throughout his memorandum books are numerous entries showing purchases of this medicine: February 21, 1778, "Pd. fr half a pound Jesuits bark," May 22, 1784, "Pd. Dr. Bass for bark 7/6," June 8,

74 J. Bear, Jr., & L. Stanton, eds., *Jefferson's Memorandum Books* (Princeton , New Jersey: Princeton University Press, Forthcoming), n.p.

75 Ibid., n.p.

1784, "Pd at Newhaven [Connecticut] for 2. oz. bark 6/." and May 1, 1790, "Pd. for 1. oz bark 3/."[76] Other entries show that Jefferson purchased gum Arabic, physic (medicine), corn salve and sulfur. It is clear that Jefferson was self-medicating, and while not unusual for his time, it highlights the fact that he was confident in his ability to treat himself and was serious about taking charge of his health care. This tendency towards self-treatment could, and probably did, instigate the home preparation and use of botanical medicines.

Further evidence of Jefferson's self-medication can be found in a brief description written by him explaining a treatment for his frequent headaches. Housed in the archives of the Library of Congress, the memorandum attests that the treatment was successful in alleviating severe head pain. Entitled "Recipe for the headach called the Sun-pain," Jefferson notes that it originated with a "drunken Doctr." who recommended it to a Mr. Willis of Georgia. The single ingredient was six grains of calomel to be taken at night and then the stomach left empty which, Jefferson states, relieved Mr. Willis of his headaches and cured Mr. Willis's son of the same ailment.[77] Jefferson recorded other instances of using calomel in attempts to relieve his headaches, though he never indicated that the treatments were successful.

Some additional and fascinating clues to Jefferson's use of medicine may lie in a small medicine box on display at Monticello. Constructed of poplar and walnut, this small chest contains eighteen empty glass vials. The most intriguing aspect of the box is the residue remaining inside the vials themselves. Two, in particular, rate special attention. The first contains a large quantity of clear crystals adhering to the inside top of the

---

76 Ibid., n.p.

77 Library of Congress Archives Document #41873.

vial. Resembling quartz crystals, they were apparently created when liquid evaporated around the glass stopper leaving a mineral residue to form on the glass. The second vial is stained by a brownish remnant. It is unknown whether the stain was left by liquid-based or solid contents. Pressing problems dealing with restoration at Monticello and the expense of testing these substances have prevented determining their identity. One day, it is to be hoped, tests will be conducted and the results will contribute an important piece to the puzzle of Jefferson's medicinal practices.

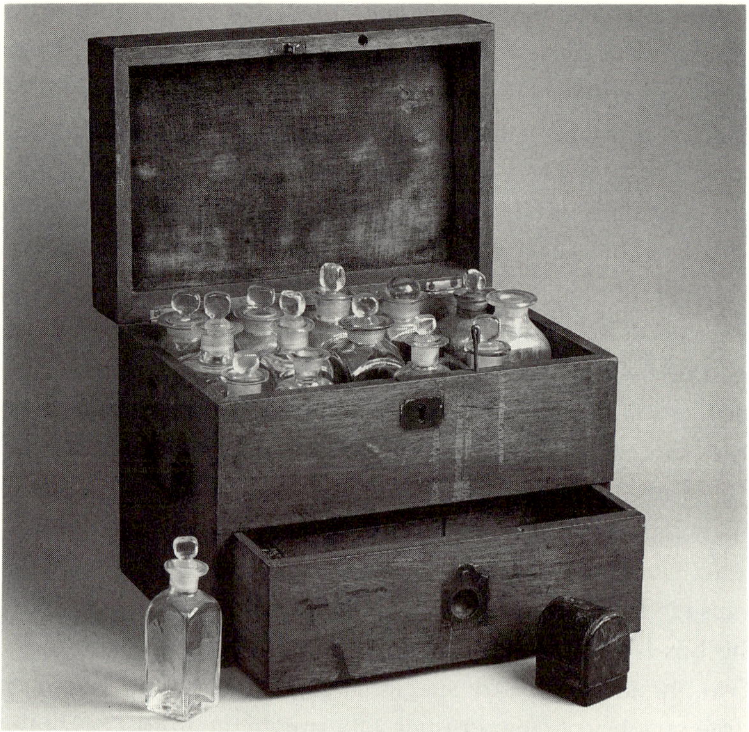

Jefferson's Medicine Box

This small poplar and walnut medicine box, on display at Monticello, still contains eighteen empty glass vials.

Courtesy of Monticello/Thomas Jefferson Memorial Foundation, Inc.

Today, individuals treat themselves with various types of over-the-counter medications. In Jefferson's day, however, equivalent medications were prepared in the kitchen or purchased from an apothecary. In either case they were often procured at the discretion of the patient and employed in the same fashion. Dosage varied with the severity of the patient's symptoms. Jefferson treated himself in the same way. He deplored the unscientific theories and practices of doctors and as a consequence was reluctant to accept their medical opinions.[78] This attitude encouraged Jefferson to seek remedies in herbs and plants. Of course, Jefferson was raised during a time when home treatment was the norm rather than the exception. Tradition and experience bolstered his efforts at therapy. With his inquisitive mind and love of plants, it is natural to infer Jefferson's use of a "garden pharmacy."

78 John D. Battle, Jr., M.D., "The 'periodical head-achs' of Thomas Jefferson," *Cleveland Clinic Quarterly* Vol. 51, No. 3 (Fall, 1984): p. 531.

CHAPTER FIVE

Jefferson on Health

I Enjoy Good Health and Spirits

Thomas Jefferson was pragmatic about his health. He believed that sustenance of good health was possible by adopting sensible health practices. His belief is manifested through personal comments on health found in a great deal of his private correspondence. He postulated strong opinions on diet, exercise, the use of alcohol and tobacco, along with outdoor and intellectual activities. Jefferson's letters illustrate his conviction that good health and quality of life are inseparable. He was emphatic whenever he mentioned the subject. Writing to his daughter, Martha, he declared, "... health is the first of all objects."[1] Jefferson recog-

1 Sarah N. Randolph, *The Domestic Life of Thomas Jefferson* (Cambridge,

nized that good health is the first priority for good living. And, for Jefferson, good living meant spending time with his family at Monticello.

Two of Thomas Jefferson's most engaging characteristics were his devotion to his family and his fascination with the natural world around him. In his letters these two features of his personality are clearly evident. He realized that both of these passions would be jeopardized if his health became seriously impaired. This realization disturbed him so much that Jefferson, the intellectual, suggested he would sacrifice knowledge before health. Writing to his son-in-law, Thomas Mann Randolph, in July 1787, Jefferson remarked, "The most uninformed mind, with a healthy body, is happier than the wisest valetudinarian," concluding "without [health] there is no happiness."[2] Jefferson perhaps gave himself up to hyperbole with the assertion that ignorance plus good health equals bliss. It does appear particularly overstated coming from the man who wrote to John Adams in June 1815, "I cannot live without books."[3] This is yet another example of the occasional lapses into contradictory statements that make Jefferson an interesting character study. There is some merit in the suggestion that Jefferson, at times, expressed opinions of convenience. For instance, when he became ill enough his stated uneasiness with physicians became secondary to the quest to reclaim his health.

Jefferson sought treatment from several doctors over his lifetime. He worried that medicine might damage his stomach, yet he took it just the same. And, while he fussed about faddish trends in medicine, he nevertheless bathed his feet in cold

---

Massachusetts: University Press, 1939), p. 86.

2 A. Koch and W. Peden, eds., *The Life and Selected Writings of Thomas Jefferson* (New York: The Modern Library, 1944), p. 426.

3 *Bartlett's Familiar Quotations,* 1992 ed., s.v. "Thomas Jefferson 1743–1826," p. 344.

water to prevent colds and rode a trotting horse in the belief that it would cure diarrhea. Jefferson protested much, but not always, apparently, with conviction.

Seeking to preserve his health, Jefferson embraced several strict habits. He was careful of his diet, he exercised, he abstained from tobacco and strong alcohol, he was outdoors whenever possible and he kept his mind active. In combination, these practices contributed to his living to the advanced age of eighty-three. Massachusetts, the only state to do so, collected life expectancy statistics for 1789. Of the males in Massachusetts that year (and, it is fair to approximate for other states, too) only fifteen percent reached the age of sixty.[4] Males, then, living to the age of eighty-three were a rare exception. Genes would not account for his longevity as his father lived only to about fifty years of age and his mother died when she was fifty-six.[5] In light of current understanding of how to preserve good health, clearly, Jefferson significantly extended his life by careful attention to wise health habits. He took good care of himself.

Jefferson was scrupulous in his diet. Vegetables, rather than meat, made up the bulk of his meals. He stated to Dr. Vine Utley in a letter dated March 21, 1819, that he was in the habit of "eating little animal food, and that not as an aliment so much as a condiment for the vegetables, which constitute my principal diet."[6] His aversion to meat and partiality for vegetables and fruits accounts for the large number of these items grown at Monticello. Jefferson was especially fond of several

---

4 R. B. and J. B. Morris, eds., *Encyclopedia of American History* (New York: Harper and Row, 1976), p. 649.

5 Dumas Malone, *Jefferson the Virginian*, vol. 1, *Jefferson and His Time* (Boston: Little, Brown and Company, 1948), p. 430.

6 A. Koch and W. Peden, eds., *The Life and Selected Writings of Thomas Jefferson* (New York: Random House, 1993), p. 631.

particular types of vegetables and fruits, which he mentions in his letters. For example, Jefferson periodically wrote of dining on salads made of lettuce, endive and other vegetables. To Anne Cary Randolph, his granddaughter, he expressed pleasure at "having a dish of sallad"[7] with his meal and to Bernard McMahon, a botanist in Philadelphia, he indicated that Monticello, to complement his salads, was producing "our own sallad oil."[8] The production of this oil sprang from the thoughtful gesture of a friend in 1807. He had sent Jefferson a sample of salad oil (produced from benne seed) which so impressed him ("I did not believe before that there existed so perfect a substitute for olive oil . . .") that he determined "to go into the culture of it for domestic use."[9] Salad became a regular part of dinner and salad oil an indispensable table item for Jefferson. His desire to have it always available is evidenced by a letter he wrote to his grandson, Thomas Jefferson Randolph, in April 1810 asking him to procure a supply quickly as "we are out of sallad-oil, and you know it is a necessary of life here . . . be particular as to its quality. If fine I would be glad to have half a dozen quarts. If absolutely not good get a single bottle only to serve till I can get some from Philadelphia."[10] The large number of lettuce plantings listed in Jefferson's *Garden Book* underscore his appreciation for various varieties of this vegetable and testify to the plentiful amounts consumed.

Cucumber was another favorite vegetable of Jefferson's. He was fond of eating them either fresh from the garden or pickled. As with so many other things at Monticello, Jefferson

---

7 Edwin Morris Betts, ed., *Thomas Jefferson's Garden Book* (Lancaster, Pennsylvania: Lancaster Press, Inc., 1944), p. 368.

8 Ibid., p. 456.

9 Ibid., p. 361.

10 E. Betts and J. Bear, Jr., eds., *The Family Letters of Thomas Jefferson* (Columbia, Missouri: University of Missouri Press, 1966), pp. 396–397.

sought to improve his cucumbers. In a letter to Thomas Worthington, Governor of Ohio, Jefferson wrote hoping that ". . . you will procure for me . . . half a dozen seeds of these mammoth cucumbers. Altho giants do not always beget giants, yet I should count on improving the breed, and this vegetable being a great favorite of mine, I wish to take the chance of an improvement."[11] Several years prior he had corresponded with his brother, Randolph Jefferson, responding to a request from their sister seeking guidance on seeds and proper planting. In the letter Jefferson carefully included "a few seeds of the Gerkin. It is that by which we distinguish the very small pickling cucumber . . . "[12] In a gesture of affection he thoughtfully enclosed a gardening book he had purchased and indexed for her so that she might "find any particular article more readily."[13]

Judging by the large number of entries for them, there were several other vegetables and fruits for which Jefferson had a particular affinity. Peas, beans, peaches and apples appear to have been among his favorites. His *Garden Book* lists many varieties of these personal preferences that were planted at Monticello.

What Jefferson considered essential to preserve his own health, he recommended to others. He was always willing, indeed seemed to feel it necessary, to share sensible ideas with neighbors and friends. It seems only fitting then to find Jefferson being consulted about a proper dietary regimen. In 1809, Jefferson responded to a letter from a gentleman in charge of a boarding house for the proposed University of Virginia. He had requested information of Jefferson pertaining to the food items

---

11 Edwin Morris Betts, ed., *Thomas Jefferson's Garden Book* (Lancaster, Pennsylvania: Lancaster Press, Inc., 1944), p. 616.

12 Ibid., p. 516.

13 Ibid.

to be served to the new students. In his reply, Jefferson set forth the following:

> for breakfast, wheat or cornbread, at the choice of each particular, with butter, and milk, or Coffee-au-lait, at the choice of each. No meat.
>
> for dinner, a soup, a dish of salt meat, a dish of fresh meat, & as great a variety of vegetables well cooked as you please.
>
> for supper, corn or wheat bread at their choice, & milk, or Coffee-au-lait, also at their choice, but no meat.[14]

Jefferson concluded his recommendations by suggesting that "their drink at all times [be] water, a young stomach needing no stimulating drinks and the habit of using them being dangerous."[15] This daily menu illustrates Jefferson's preference for vegetables over meat. His concession to meat for dinner was offset by the inclusion, at the same time, of a large number of vegetables. Apparently, he thought that the large variety of vegetables would distract a diner's attention from the meat. His admonition against serving alcohol will be taken up later.

It is clear from his dietary practices and advice that Jefferson was a proponent of health maintenance. He both practiced and promoted his philosophy of health preservation to avoid the more difficult problem of health restoration. This was not a novelty for Jefferson but a lifelong commitment.

The contents of Jefferson's library testified to the seriousness with which he approached his health. His thousands of volumes, covering scores of topics, included a large number of works on health maintenance. Among these were: *Hills Old Man's Guide* (*The Old Man's Guide to Health and Longer Life*:

14 A. Koch and W. Peden, eds., *The Life and Selected Writings of Thomas Jefferson* (New York: Random House, 1993), p. 632.

15 Ibid.

with rules for Diet, Exercise, and Physic, for preserving a good Constitution, and Preventing Disorders in a bad one) written by Sir John Hill, *Peale on the Means of Preserving Health* written by Charles Willson Peale, *Ricketson's Means of Preserving Health* by Shadrach Ricketson and *Baynard on Cold Bathing* authored by Edward Baynard.[16] This last work encouraged a peculiar habit of Jefferson's as evidenced by his letter to James Maury in June 1815,

> I have for 50. years bathed my feet in cold water every morning . . . and have been remarkably exempted from colds (not having had one in every 7. years of my life on an average) I have supposed it might be ascribed to that practice. When we see two facts accompanying one another for a long time we are apt to suppose them related as cause and effect.[17]

Jefferson was quite convinced that bathing his feet in cold water was responsible for his having had few colds. Despite his obvious faith in the merits of this practice it seems that he did not make a point of recommending it to others. In his letter to the University of Virginia landlord discussing daily meal items he had included a directive that no "stimulating drink" be allowed, but he had not included one insisting that the young men likewise bathe their feet in cold water to prevent colds.[18]

It can be inferred that Jefferson clearly saw a vice in alcohol but, despite his cause and effect assessment, not as clearly a virtue in cold water therapy.

Thomas Jefferson did, however, believe that there was virtue in habitual exercise. His letters frequently address the issue of exercising the body, and he took every opportunity to

---

16 E. Millicent Sowerby, ed., *Catalogue of the Library of Thomas Jefferson* (Unknown: The Library of Congress, 1952), pp. 415–417.

17 Ibid., p. 417.

18 A. Koch and W. Peden, eds., *The Life and Selected Writings of Thomas Jefferson* (New York: Random House, 1993), p. 632.

encourage this habit in family members. Jefferson enjoyed walks and took particular pleasure in horseback riding. Sarah Randolph, Jefferson's granddaughter, recalled that Jefferson had a "custom of taking regular daily exercise" and that "he never failed . . . no matter what his occupation, to devote the hours between one and three in the afternoon to exercise, which was most frequently taken on horseback."[19] Jefferson's enjoyment of riding horseback remained with him through the final days of his life. Thomas Jefferson Randolph recalled, "he retained to the last his fondness for riding on horseback; he rode within three weeks of his death, when from disease, debility and age, he mounted with difficulty."[20]

In a letter written by Jefferson to his nephew, Peter Carr, he expressed an equal enthusiasm for walking. He told his nephew, "walking is the best possible exercise. Habituate yourself to walk very far."[21] Jefferson's advice to his nephew is a prime example of his forward thinking. Jefferson was right, of course. Contemporary research has demonstrated that regular extended brisk walks contribute significantly to good health. A granddaughter of Jefferson's told Jefferson biographer Henry Randall that her grandfather believed strongly in walking and "every day he . . . walked in his garden."[22] His daughter, Martha, summed up Jefferson's appreciation for both types of exercise when she stated that while residing in Paris, "he always rode or walked as far as seven miles into the country."[23] Exercise was a valued part of Jefferson's daily routine. Expressing

---

19 Sarah N. Randolph, *The Domestic Life of Thomas Jefferson* (Cambridge, Massachusetts: University Press, 1939), pp. 246–247.

20 Ibid., p. 289.

21 A. Koch and W. Peden, eds., *The Life and Selected Writings of Thomas Jefferson* (New York: Random House, 1993), p. 349.

22 Sarah N. Randolph, *The Domestic Life of Thomas Jefferson* (Cambridge, Massachusetts: University Press, 1939), p. 292.

23 Ibid., p. 48.

his belief in its worth, Jefferson wrote Martha, "exercise and application produce order in our affairs, health of body, cheerfulness of mind, and these make us precious to our friends."[24]

Jefferson believed, as well, in exercising the mind and conscience of the individual. "A mind always employed is always happy. This is the true secret, the general recipe, for felicity."[25] Jefferson considered reading one of the best ways of employing the mind. He told Carr that when studying Moral Philosophy ". . . read good books, because they will encourage, as well as direct your feelings."[26] As for his nephew's conscience, Jefferson told him, "The moral sense, or conscience, is as much a part of man as his leg or arm. It may be strengthened by exercise, as may any particular limb of the body" and that exercise of the conscience occurs when one endeavors "to be grateful, to be generous, to be charitable, to be humane, to be true, just, firm, orderly, courageous, & c."[27] In short, Carr was to develop his honor and integrity by applying them.

Thomas Jefferson, owner of thousands of books, quite obviously appreciated the benefits of reading. His observations on what constituted a happy mind and a strong conscience were based on learning and experience. Jefferson displayed prescience with his emphasis on mental health, comprehending the importance of its role in daily living. The ideas for health and happiness that Jefferson formulated and refined over his lifetime constituted a well balanced program of mental, moral and physical pursuits. His exhortations to his family to follow these precepts were born of an understanding of their

---

24 E. Betts and J. Bear, Jr., eds., *The Family Letters of Thomas Jefferson* (Columbia, Missouri: University of Missouri Press, 1966), p. 34.

25 Sarah N. Randolph, *The Domestic Life of Thomas Jefferson* (Cambridge, Massachusetts: University Press, 1939), p. 93.

26 A. Koch and W. Peden, eds., *The Life and Selected Writings of Thomas Jefferson* (New York: Random House, 1993), p. 398.

27 Ibid., pp. 398–399.

importance to a wholesome lifestyle. Jefferson had a distinct awareness of the hebetude that separates individuals from an active or sedentary lifestyle and the end results of each. He was not one for idleness; physical and mental exercise became second nature to him and, in conjunction with his abstinence from tobacco and hard spirits, also became daily patterns which enhanced his chances of staying healthy.

Besides his horseback riding and walking, Jefferson also participated in other outdoor activities. According to Sarah Randolph, Jefferson's father, Peter Jefferson, believing physical exercise to be part of a young man's development, had taught his son to swim when he was an adolescent.[28] In addition, while at college, Jefferson enjoyed running from town "to a certain stone which stood at a point a mile beyond" and back again.[29] It was in the fresh air, she said, where ". . . he found his favorite recreations in out-of-doors enjoyments. . . . "[30]

Another outdoor activity that Jefferson enjoyed immensely was gardening. His *Garden Book*, begun when he was in his early twenties, testifies to his passion for planting and growing all types of plants. By the time he moved to Monticello, he had observed gardens of varying sophistication along with the art of gardening and was an experienced gardener himself.[31] He enjoyed gardening for the healthful benefits of fresh air. To Martha, who at the time was recovering from an illness, he once wrote, "I hope you are getting well, towards which great care of yourself is necessary. You will be out in time to begin your garden and that will tempt you to be

---

28 Sarah N. Randolph, *The Domestic Life of Thomas Jefferson* (Cambridge, Massachusetts: University Press, 1939), p. 6.

29 Ibid., p. 15.

30 Ibid., p. 29.

31 E. M. Betts and H. B. Perkins, *Thomas Jefferson's Flower Garden at Monticello* (Charlottesville, Virginia: University of Virginia Press, 1986), p. 2.

out a great deal, than which nothing will tend more to give you health and strength."[32]

Jefferson was as earnest about gardening as an art as he was about gardening for the sake of health. As evidence of the high esteem in which he held this pastime, in 1814 he proposed that gardening be taught in the Fine Arts Department of the planned University of Virginia along with architecture, painting, sculpture and music.[33] He perceived thoroughly that gardening was salutary for the mind as well as the body.

Apparently recognizing that tobacco use is unhealthy, Jefferson shied away from the weed. Not a single instance has been found where he stated, or where it is documented by others, that he used tobacco. Although Jefferson, like many Virginians, grew tobacco, he evidently had a personal aversion to it. Jefferson's biographer, Dumas Malone, states that without exception, "he [Jefferson] did not use tobacco."[34] Being a health conscious individual he must have sensed an inherent danger in its use. His insight was too keen to miss its hazards. Yet, it was a money making crop, and while he might not risk its use, he had no compunction against raising and selling it for others to use. He did not indulge in it, and he could have spoken out against its use, but it generated money and money added a certain convenience to living. As with certain other issues, Jefferson is again discovered in a contradiction.

Jefferson perceived wine, however, quite differently. He had a great deal of veneration for it, if only the weaker varieties. Many of these less vigorous wines he believed to be restor-

---

32 E. Betts and J. Bear, Jr., eds., *The Family Letters of Thomas Jefferson* (Columbia, Missouri: University of Missouri Press, 1966), pp. 71–72.

33 A. Koch and W. Peden, eds., *The Life and Selected Writings of Thomas Jefferson* (New York: Random House, 1993), p. 591.

34 Dumas Malone, *Jefferson the President*, vol. 4, *Jefferson and His Time* (Boston: Little, Brown and Company, 1970), p. 186.

atives. The more potent wines he avoided altogether in keeping with his objection to strong drink. To Dr. Utley, Jefferson wrote in 1819, "the ardent wines I cannot drink, nor do I use ardent spirits in any form."[35] Thomas Jefferson Randolph tells us that "such was his aversion . . . that when, in his last illness, his physician desired him to use brandy as an astringent, he could not induce him to take it strong enough."[36] Jefferson did, as noted, believe weaker wines to be beneficial to health and digestion and, as such, he promoted their use among his family members. To his ailing daughter, Mary Jefferson Eppes, he had recommended the use of "light food and cordial wines" along with a "Pedro Ximenes" as a stomachic with which to cure her fever.[37]

In a letter written to a Portuguese wine merchant in 1815, Jefferson said, "wine from long habit has become an indispensable for my health, which is now suffering by its desire" and, in keeping with his dislike of strong wines, added, "[Madeira] is a wine which I do not drink being entirely too powerful."[38] Jefferson considered the use of light wines an integral part of his health care program.

Jefferson kept the cellars of Monticello well-stocked. In anticipation of his return home in August 1793, he wrote Martha, "I received information yesterday of 500 bottles of wine arrived for me at Baltimore. I desired them to be . . . forwarded to Monticello."[39] Having a well-stocked wine cellar was essen-

---

35 A. Koch and W. Peden, eds., *The Life and Selected Writings of Thomas Jefferson* (New York: Random House, 1993), p. 631.

36 Sarah N. Randolph, *The Domestic Life of Thomas Jefferson* (Cambridge, Massachusetts: University Press, 1939), p. 290.

37 Ibid., p. 255.

38 Lawrence R. de Treville, III, *Jefferson and Wine: Model of Moderation* (The Plains, Virginia: Vinifera Wine Growers Assoc., 1989), p. 103.

39 E.Betts and J. Bear, Jr., eds., *The Family Letters of Thomas Jefferson* (Columbia, Missouri: University of Missouri Press, 1966), p. 123.

tial for a man of refinement and, for Jefferson, a medicinal necessity as well.

Jefferson made it his habit to consume wine each day. When comparing his daily usage to that of his good friend Dr. Rush, Jefferson wrote, "I double . . . the Doctor's glass and a half of wine, and even treble it with a friend; but halve its effect by drinking the weak wines only."[40] Jefferson felt little need or inclination to drink water; Colonel Jefferson Randolph, stated that "he drank water but once a day, a single glass, when he returned from his ride."[41] Jefferson's bias and liking for wine was plain; it was his drink of preference and he encouraged its consumption, telling Monsieur de Neuville in 1818 that "its extended use will carry health and comfort to a much enlarged circle. . . ."[42] It would not surprise Jefferson to learn that a recent European study has shown that routine moderate use of wine may reduce the chances of a heart attack and lower serum cholesterol levels.

Thomas Jefferson enjoyed a lifetime of few serious illnesses. Most certainly his personal health habits contributed to this overall good health. It is a now established fact that proper diet and exercise can assist in maintaining health and increase the prospects of living longer. Framed against a backdrop of modern medical knowledge, Jefferson's lifestyle takes on a twentieth-century appearance. Jefferson did not, however, escape his share of lesser illnesses. His troublesome headaches and years of periodic diarrhea are examples of less serious, but vexatious, ailments from which he suffered. And, despite his

---

40 A. Koch and W. Peden, eds., *The Life and Selected Writings of Thomas Jefferson* (New York: Random House, 1993), p. 631.

41 Sarah N. Randolph, *The Domestic Life of Thomas Jefferson* (Cambridge, Massachusetts: University Press, 1939), p. 290.

42 Lawrence R. de Treville, III, *Jefferson and Wine: Model of Moderation* (The Plains, Virginia: Vinifera Wine Growers Assoc., 1989), p. 288.

cold water foot baths, he did contract a head cold from time to time. A letter to Martha sent from Philadelphia in 1792 told her "I was prevented writing to you last week by a bad cold attended with fever. . . .[43] In 1797, writing again from Philadelphia, Jefferson informed her "I am at length got well of a terrible cold . . . it is now entirely passed off."[44]

For a man to live to beyond eighty years of age in Jefferson's day was an attainment worthy of note. As indicated previously, only a small percentage lived to the age of sixty. Considered in that context, colds, headaches and an irritable bowel left Jefferson little room for complaint. And, in fact, he did not complain. In describing his health over his life time he said,

> I have been more fortunate than my friend [Dr. Rush] in the article of health. So free from catarrhs that I have not had one, (in the breast, I mean) on an average of eight or ten years through life. A fever of more than twenty-four hours I have not had above two or three times in my life. A periodical headache has afflicted me occasionally . . . I enjoy good health.[45]

Jefferson's own evaluation of his health fails to mention his diarrhea. Did he consider this problem to be of too personal a nature? Did he believe the condition to be something other than a physical ailment? Might Jefferson have considered this malady psychological? He may have perceived a correlation between the stress of governmental life and his bowel irregularities and concluded that his diarrhea was, in fact, a manifestation of the rigors of being a public figure.

---

43 E. Betts and J. Bear, Jr., eds., *The Family Letters of Thomas Jefferson* (Columbia, Missouri: University of Missouri Press, 1966), p. 93.

44 Ibid., p.150.

45 A. Koch and W. Peden, eds., *The Life and Selected Writings of Thomas Jefferson* (New York: Random House, 1993), p. 631.

Consider a letter written by Jefferson to Henry Fry of Madison County, Virginia. Jefferson wrote Fry that a trotting horse strengthens the bowels and would aid Fry in arresting his diarrhea, adding that he had used the treatment himself, suggested by the British physician, Dr. Thomas Sydenham, and believed that it had cured him (it had not).[46] It is puzzling that someone with Jefferson's mental acumen could have convinced himself that a cure existed in such a fanciful treatment. Conceivably, Jefferson's horseback riding brought about much needed relaxation, which in turn, resulted in a temporary cessation of his diarrhea. An understanding of stress and its health implications would wait for a later age, but Jefferson's subconscious may well have preempted the findings of future mental health research. Of course, the explanation may be simpler than that. His foot baths are a reminder that Jefferson could be drawn to odd indulgences and was not above engaging in faddish treatments. The trotting horse "remedy" could be a case in point.

The record of Jefferson's health supports his statements that overall he enjoyed a life free of serious health impairments. This can be attributed to his diet, regular exercise, abstinence from tobacco and strong drink and simple good luck. He escaped exposure to nearly all of the lethal illnesses prevalent during his lifetime: diphtheria, typhoid, yellow fever, small pox (he had been inoculated) and pneumonia. Jefferson no doubt would have credited his escape from this last disease to his daily cold water foot bath. He was convinced that this odd habit could do for him what medicine could not, declaring to Dr. Henry Wheaton that he had "little confidence in the theories of

46 E. Millicent Sowerby, *Catalogue of the Library of Thomas Jefferson* (Unknown: The Library of Congress, 1952), p. 411.

that Art [medicine], which change in their fashion with the ladies caps and gowns. . . ."[47]

Jefferson is said to have been afflicted with only two potentially deadly illnesses during his life—dysentery and tuberculosis. In a monograph on Jefferson's health written by James A. Bear, Jr. and Gordon Jones, M.D., the authors state that Jefferson became ill with dysentery as a young man while a member of the Virginia House of Burgesses.[48] They further contend that he was a victim of tuberculosis and suffered with it from late 1783 until 1786 after which "if we except his troubles with his broken wrist, Jefferson had few ailments."[49]

Conjuring up a mental image of Jefferson with his feet immersed in cold water baths to prevent colds or bouncing about on horseback to cure diarrhea elicits a smile. Perhaps at no other time does he appear so human and so like an ordinary man. In truth, Jefferson saw himself as perfectly average, telling his friend Dr. Vine Utley, "I live so much like other people, that I might refer to ordinary life as the history of my own . . . my life has been so much like that of other people, that I might say . . . *nomine mutato, narratur fabula de te* [with a change of name, the tale can be told of you]."[50]

Jefferson's diarrhea and headaches were, of course, uncomfortable, and at times incapacitating, but never life threatening. Many of Jefferson's contemporaries suffered with similar ailments and, like Jefferson, learned to live with them. Then, as now, the odds of experiencing a lifetime free of injury or disease were astronomical. Injuries, diseases and their con-

---

47 Ibid., p. 446.

48 J.A. Bear, Jr. and G. Jones, M.D., *Thomas Jefferson and His Health* (None: Unpublished, None), p. 5.

49 Ibid.

50 A. Koch and W. Peden, eds., *The Life and Selected Writings of Thomas Jefferson* (New York: Random House, 1993), pp. 631–632.

sequences were inevitable. It may have been Jefferson's familiarity with the physical condition of many of his contemporaries that prompted his assertion of overall personal good health. In comparing himself with his acquaintances, he may have realized that he experienced fewer ailments. Or it could be that with his optimistic perspective on life, he was determined not to allow illness to detract from its joys. More than likely, a combination of these factors, coupled with the personal health habits that he had practiced during his life, let him recognize and enjoy his superior physical condition.

Jefferson's viewpoint on living and illness are best expressed in a letter to William Short written at Monticello, October 31, 1819. In the letter Jefferson chides Short for his capitulation to indolence telling him, "your love of repose will lead, in its progress to a suspension of healthy exercise, a relaxation of the mind, an indifference to everything around you, and finally to a debility of body, and hebetude of mind. . . ."[51]

His "philosophy of living," proper diet, exercise, abstinence from tobacco and strong drink, and scholarship enabled Jefferson to enjoy a long and relatively healthy life. As he approached his twilight years, Jefferson was determined to retain his involvement in those established activities which had so enriched him. At age seventy-five he reported to Dr. Benjamin Waterhouse that although he was declining in body and memory "still, however, I enjoy good health and spirits, and am as industrious a reader as when a student at college. . . ."[52]

Indolence would never claim Thomas Jefferson as an acquaintance.

51 Ibid., pp. 634–635.

52 Ibid., p. 627.

CHAPTER SIX

Health Is the First Requisite

A Jefferson Legacy

AMERICANS INHERITED A NUMBER OF LEGACIES FROM Thomas Jefferson. Probably the least known and understood is that of health preservation. Jefferson thought the maintenance of health was a matter of personal responsibility as well as a requisite of good citizenship. In his mind it was a simple matter to connect good personal health with the nation's health. Healthy citizens are necessary for a sound nation. Only healthy citizens can maintain a vibrant and robust government. The fitness of the country's democratic institutions is proportional to the hardiness of its people. Sound health must be a personal priority. To his nephew, Thomas Mann Randolph, Jr., he wrote in 1787, "an attention to health . . . should take the place of every other object. The time necessary to secure this . . . should be devoted to it in preference to every other pursuit."[1] In other words, whatever the time required or the pursuit postponed, an individual's first priority must be good health.

1 A. Koch and W. Peden, eds., *The Life and Selected Writings of Thomas Jefferson* (New York: Random House, 1993), p. 394.

John M. Dorsey, M.D. summed up Jefferson's philosophy on health in his work, *The Jefferson-Dunglison Letters*. Dr. Dorsey wrote that Jefferson,

> recognized that healing must occur in the one to be healed, not in his physician or in the no man's land between each individual; that each sick man must be his own patient as well as his own physician; that no individual can delegate his healing power to another person any more than to his State. As the individual is the guardian of all of his liberty, so must he also guard his own healing power, therapy being a part of his nature.[2]

Dorsey captured the essence of Thomas Jefferson, his unqualified belief in the supremacy of the individual and his conviction that the strength of America lay in the individualism of its people; an individualism reflected in the recognition of the right to heal oneself, to be assertive in the pursuit of health care, to seek dominion over the fashion of treatment and never to surrender the right of decision-making towards personal well-being, as one should never surrender any other right.

Jefferson was determined to hold sway over his health. He read, he questioned and he thought. He leaned heavily on his distrust of physicians and his belief that if left alone, the body would care for itself. Indeed, Jefferson did occasionally consult doctors. Always, however, this was a latter alternative and not an initial step.

In Jefferson's well founded opinion, the medical profession of his day had barely begun to comprehend the complexities of the body and the causes of disease.[3]

As a consequence, it warrants restating, his relationships

2 John M. Dorsey, M.D., ed., *The Jefferson-Dunglison Letters* (Charlottesville, Virginia: University of Virginia Press, 1960), p. 93.

3 Dumas Malone, *Jefferson the President*, vol. 4, *Jefferson and His Time* (Boston: Little, Brown and Company, 1970), p. 184.

with physicians were most often personal and intellectual rather than professional. Jefferson's primary interest in medicine lay in the study of it.

Jefferson was fully aware that an individual must not surrender the care of one's health to another. To do so would be to abrogate a fundamental responsibility. That being the moral imperative a free citizen of America assumes in order to honor and fulfill the precepts of the Declaration of Independence. The rights of life, liberty and the pursuit of happiness rest on our physical well being. These rights cannot be enjoyed by citizens who sacrifice their health. In the absence of good health these rights are rendered moot.

Further, in a democracy it is the responsibility of individuals to exercise their rights, including the right to act as one's own physician. Free people must approach medicine with a healthy amount of skepticism. They must be willing to question and disagree and to demand equal involvement in any decision regarding treatment. In sum they must never relinquish the right of control over their health.

Throughout his lifetime Jefferson exercised his right to act as his own doctor. Contained in his health ideology was the view that by nature man seeks to treat himself. He acts to throw off the shackles of disease as naturally as those of tyranny. Jefferson valued this right of self-care as much as any other. And, surely he was committed to the concept that he who accepts responsibility for his health takes pleasure in his health.

Jefferson was tolerant of medicine only as far as evidence would take it. On one occasion, writing to Benjamin Rush, he declared "... I acknowledge facts in medicine as far as they go, distrusting only their extension by theory."[4]

4 A. Koch and W. Peden, eds., *The Life and Selected Writings of Thomas Jefferson* (New York: Random House, 1993), p. 562.

It was when physicians pressed treatment beyond the point of their knowledge and experience that Jefferson protested most vigorously. Had Jefferson been aware of it, he might have used as an example the treatment George Washington received during his final illness. In the span of a few short hours, Washington was bled four times, dosed three times with calomel and once with tartar emetic and his throat was blistered with Spanish fly.[5]

Washington's doctors were treating an illness which they could barely comprehend, much less knowledgeably minister to. His illness quickly out-distanced his doctor's professional abilities and in their desperation to do something, anything, they only added to their patient's torment. Washington's horrific treatment was the sort that Jefferson had denounced as inhumane. He was firmly committed to limited therapy; the rest and best of the cure was then left to nature.

Jefferson was capable of subordinating his convictions to suit his purpose if he believed that circumstances warranted such a turn. In a letter to Peter Carr dated August 10, 1787, Jefferson wrote, "health is the first requisite after morality."[6]

This was not the opinion Jefferson had expressed to others when he explained that health was always to be placed first. Something had altered Jefferson's priorities. Carr was by this time a young adult and, perhaps, Jefferson was taking the opportunity to impress upon his nephew the importance of righteous living. This is an intriguing possibility in that certain members of Jefferson's family, and some later historians, have suggested that Carr may have fathered the children of Sally Hemings (one of Jefferson's slaves). Jefferson may well have

---

5 Richard Norton Smith, *Patriarch* (Boston: Houghton Mifflin Company, 1993), p. 353.

6 A. Koch and W. Peden, eds., *The Life and Selected Writings of Thomas Jefferson* (New York: Random House, 1993), p. 401.

perceived in young Carr a propensity for promiscuous behavior.

In the same letter to Carr is a startling command from Jefferson which illustrates his phobia of accepting nothing without reasoned evaluation. He wrote to Carr, "question with boldness even the existence of a God."[7] A man who would dispense a directive such as this certainly would not hesitate to question a physician. In fact, he would do so eagerly, enjoying the process and with less chance of damnation!

Jefferson's attitude with most doctors was essentially the same as that which he showed toward Benjamin Rush. When writing him about his diarrhea, Jefferson, in anticipation of a reply respecting a treatment, "made it perfectly clear that he wanted fact, not theories."[8] He was disappointed. When a lengthy response from Rush arrived, Jefferson read the doctor's numerous recommended treatments, then wrote thanking him, but closed the letter saying, "I shall with confidence avail myself of [your] general prescriptions and of the special [one] should the state of my health alter for the *worse*."[9] As uncomfortable as he was, he perceived rashness in Rush's prescribed treatments of powder of oak gall with cinnamon and blistering of his wrists and ankles.[10] Jefferson obviously had hoped that Rush might suggest a remedy that was at least plausible. The advice that he received, his common sense told him, was frivolous. Although he respected and liked Rush, Jefferson would not engage in what he deemed to be farcical remedies.

Jefferson's ability to recognize his health needs and his

---

7 Ibid., p. 399.

8 Dumas Malone, *Jefferson the President*, vol. 4, *Jefferson and His Time* (Boston: Little, Brown and Company, 1970), p. 186.

9 James A. Bear, Jr., *Unpublished medical chronology of Thomas Jefferson.* Monticello Research Archives, n.d., p. 646.

10 Ibid., p. 645.

desire to seek responsible remedies underscores his passion for free thinking. He placed great hope in a future where individuals were skilled in critical thinking. Questioning, gathering facts, scrutinizing, then deciding a course of action—these were the processes he went through in all of his affairs. Certainly, his health owed much to this strict attention.

Jefferson harbored hard feelings for physicians who used violent therapeutic measures to treat patients. Scarifying the flesh to bleed, administering harsh drugs for violent vomiting and employing wolfish medications against the bowels disturbed Jefferson greatly. He found barbarous a physician's willingness to employ these tortures with little if any benefit to the patient. There is no evidence that this so-called heroic medicine was ever used on Jefferson. He was aware of its frightful application and judged it better suited to quacks. Proper diet, exercise and reliance on the beneficence of nature were Jefferson's treatments of choice.

When Dr. Robley Dunglison left England to accept a faculty position at the University of Virginia it was not fully for the purpose of training future physicians. The intent was to provide the University's students with enough information to enable them to fully appreciate the shortcomings of the art of healing.[11] In other words, Dunglison's responsibility was to teach the inadequacies of his chosen profession. As a result of his attitude toward the field of medicine, Jefferson insisted on providing the students with courses that would give them a true picture of medical practice.

In spite of Jefferson's misgivings about doctors and, no doubt, prompted by concern for his declining health, he invited Dr. Dunglison to act as his personal physician. Dunglison

11 John M. Dorsey, M.D., ed., *The Jefferson-Dunglison Letters* (Charlottesville, Virginia: University of Virginia Press, 1960), pp. 74–75.

treated Jefferson for less than two years. The two men quickly discovered, however, that they held a great deal in common. Dunglison, like his patient, realized that the practice of medicine left a great deal to be desired. This belief was openly displayed not long after Jefferson's death when a serious epidemic struck the University of Virginia, claiming the lives of several students. In the aftermath, Dunglison wrote an article in which he stated that physicians "are totally unacquainted with the cause of every endemic and epidemic disease of every kind."[12] Jefferson would have applauded the doctor's assessment of medicine's ignorance. He might, however, have been too modest to agree with the good doctor's assessment of him personally, "he [Jefferson] was kind, courteous, hospitable to all; I had the most exalted opinion of him. I believed him essentially a philanthropist, anxious for the greatest good to the greatest number; a distinguished patriot . . . who was eminently virtuous with fixed and honorable principles of action."[13] It was Dunglison who eventually convinced the trustees to expand the scope of the School of Medicine. Two years after Jefferson's death, the first Doctor of Medicine degrees were conferred at the University of Virginia.[14]

A final look at the Jefferson-Dunglison relationship helps underscore Jefferson's attitude toward personal health care. Dunglison had received an urgent summons to Monticello for consultation and, upon arriving at Jefferson's bedside, quickly determined that Jefferson was dying. Jefferson, exercising his right of final authority, expressed his agreement with the doctor's prognosis by not "indulg[ing] in any other opinion."[15]

---

12 Ibid., p. 77.

13 Ibid., pp. 89–90.

14 Ibid., p. 75.

15 E. Betts and J. Bear, Jr., eds., *The Family Letters of Thomas Jefferson* (Columbia, Missouri: University of Missouri Press, 1966), p. 479.

In Jefferson's mind the physician and patient relationship, to the end, should be one of ultimate concordance.

Jefferson's interest in botany was noted earlier. His fascination with the subject is reflected in the wide variety of flowers, herbs, fruits and grains grown at Monticello. He recorded when and where they were planted, he monitored their growth patterns and studied the insects and diseases that attacked them. It necessarily follows then, that he also had an interest in the medicinal potential of his plants. Jefferson's involvement with botanical remedies highlights the role that they have played throughout history. Many of our earliest ancestors concocted "cures" from herbs and plants. While most of these withered under the glare of scientific scrutiny, others were found to be valid and valuable. More importantly, new drugs from plants emerged from this research. The world of plants has given us digitalis from the foxglove, opium (morphine and codeine) from the poppy, steroids from *Dioscorea* (a yam from Mexico) and the "wonder drug" aspirin (acetylsalicylic acid) from the leaves of the plant *Spiraea Ulmaria.*[16] Today, scientists continue to search the world over for plants that may give us tomorrow's wonder drugs. In this search for new medicines Jefferson would be among the first to support investigating the botanical world. Today's scientists can derive inspiration from Jefferson's faith in the benefits of plants.

Jefferson continually experimented with plants and received a constant supply of seeds and seedlings from friends in America and in Europe. Noted American horticulturist, Bernard McMahon, of Philadelphia, corresponded with Jefferson for years, each man frequently sending packets of seeds to the other. Jefferson sent McMahon many of the plants and seeds

16 Norman Taylor, *Plant Drugs that Changed the World* (New York: Dodd, Mead & Company, 1965), pp. 123–238 passim.

returned by the Lewis and Clark expedition.[17] Andre Thouin, the famous French botanist, periodically sent Jefferson massive numbers of seeds. Jefferson wrote Martha in October of 1808, "... my old friend Thouin of the National Garden at Paris has sent me 700. species of seeds."[18]

Jefferson delighted in the opportunity to cultivate new plants. To him, planting and growing were labors of love. In a letter dated 1811 to Charles Willson Peale he wrote,

> I have often thought that if heaven had given me choice of my position and calling, it should have been a rich spot of earth, well watered, and near a good market for the productions of the garden. No occupation is so delightful to me as the cultivation of the earth, and no culture comparable to that of the garden ... I am still devoted to the garden. But though as old man, I am but a young gardener.[19]

He possessed a passion for studying all types of living things and he wrote detailed reports of his observations. His reverential enthusiasm for nature is revealed in a letter to daughter Mary written from Philadelphia, March 31, 1791,

> I wrote you in my last that the frogs had begun their songs on the 7th. Since that the blue-birds saluted us on the 17th; the weeping-willow began to leaf on the 18th; the lilac and gooseberry on the 25th; and the golden-willow on the 26th. I enclose for your sister three kinds of flowering beans, very beautiful and very rare. She must plant and nourish them with her own hand this year, in order to save enough seeds for herself and me.[20]

---

17 Edwin Morris Betts, ed., *Thomas Jefferson's Garden Book* (Lancaster, Pennsylvania: Lancaster press, Inc., 1944), p. 313–314.

18 E. Betts and J. Bear, Jr., eds., *The Family Letters of Thomas Jefferson* (Columbia, Missouri: University of Missouri Press, 1966), p. 351.

19 E. M. Betts and H. B. Perkins, *Thomas Jefferson's Flower Garden at Monticello* (Charlottesville, Virginia: University of Virginia Press, 1986), p. 20.

20 E. Betts and J. Bear, Jr., eds., *The Family Letters of Thomas Jefferson* (Columbia, Missouri: University of Missouri Press, 1966), p. 77.

It was his infatuation with nature in general that inspired Jefferson to seek out "very beautiful and very rare" plants and propagate their species. What aroused his greatest interest, however, was the work to be done to determine and promulgate the hardiest varieties of those plants that provided food and medicine. For it was with these that individuals might insure better health.

Health was never far from Jefferson's mind, either his own or his family's. To Martha he expressed his continual concern for the welfare of his loved ones: "experience leads us to be always anxious about the health of those whom we love."[21] Experience had led Jefferson all too well. He had lost his beloved wife, Martha, three infant children and was still to suffer the loss of his youngest daughter, Mary Jefferson Eppes. In the most personally painful manner imaginable, Jefferson learned the precariousness of health and the fragility of life.

Because of these tragic losses of family members, Jefferson seems to have developed a sense of urgency towards living. Every waking moment was filled with some sort of activity. Jefferson explained to Thaddeus Koscuisko, a former army officer who had served under George Washington, that from morning to evening he worked about his farms and from "dinner to dark, I give to society and recreation . . . and from candle light to early bed-time, I read."[22] This regimen, he believed, led him to enjoy "perfect health" and considerable strength.[23]

Jefferson's active and studious lifestyle, was to him, the ideal blend of the physical and mental exercise necessary for a sound body and mind. Perhaps it also served to help suppress the memories of death in his mind, as well as keep its clutches from his body.

---

21 A. Koch and W. Peden, eds., *The Life and Selected Writings of Thomas Jefferson* (New York: Random House, 1993), p. 388.

22 Ibid., p. 552.

23 Ibid.

Thomas Jefferson was a model for self-thinking. He understood that his intellect was a powerful asset, and he used it. Questioning his physician, perusing his medical references and prescribing self-therapy were all parts of his health plan. Having good health, Jefferson knew, required that he take an active role. Good health did not depend on the doctor; it was his individual responsibility.

He gave equal consideration to both his mental and physical health. He recognized the link between a sound mind and a sound body. This was not an innovative concept of Jefferson's. He read ancient history. He was aware of the Greek devotion to mental and physical exercise to strengthen thought and deed. Jefferson characterized his sentiments concerning a healthy mind in the following manner:

> For thus I estimate the qualities of the mind:
> 1. good humor;
> 2. integrity;
> 3. industry;
> 4. science;
>
> The preference of the first to the second quality may not at first be acquiesced in; but certainly we had all rather associate with a good-humored, light-principled man, than with an ill-tempered rigorist in morality.[24]

Jefferson understood that good physical health begins with the mind. It is the seat of reason and understanding. Focusing his efforts, he developed a program of individualized health care and mental verve. Jefferson's program required putting thoughts into action, enabling the mind to direct behavior. The mind conceived worthwhile health habits; the body carried them out and benefited.

---

24 John M. Dorsey, M.D., ed., *The Jefferson-Dunglison Letters* (Charlottesville, Virginia: University of Virginia Press, 1960), p. 100.

The results of these efforts would be lessened, however, if there were no physicians properly trained to operate in partnership with the individual. It was Jefferson's hope that medicine would one day move from fantasy to fact. The finest doctor could rank no higher than the lowest charlatan if his knowledge consisted solely of whimsical theories. To Dr. Caspar Wistar, Jefferson wrote in 1807,

> I wish to see a reform, an abandonment of hypothesis for sober facts, the first degree of value set on clinical observation, and the lowest on visionary theories. The only sure foundations of medicine are, an intimate knowledge of the human body, and observation on the effects of medicinal substances on that.[25]

Whatever faith Jefferson had held in medicine vanished with the deaths of his wife and children. It could not withstand the realities of loved ones lost, or his blistering scrutiny which followed. Medicine's deceits were to him mischievous and potentially fatal. The only solutions, as he indicated to Wistar, were study and research. Medicine could not advance until rigid standards of learning were applied to it. Working with the human body, Jefferson made clear, demanded a detailed understanding of its systems and a complete comprehension of applied drugs.

The medicinal material of Jefferson's time is dwarfed by the quantity and sophistication of medications available today. Phenomenal advances in medical research have ushered in an era of organ transplants and wonder drugs. Jefferson would be awed but gratified were he to see the vast changes that have evolved in the practice of medicine. Rigorous instruction and clinical training, both of which Jefferson advocated, have turned physicians into highly-trained professionals. In conjunc-

---

25 Ibid., pp. 103–104.

tion, aggressive drug research continues to expand our pharmacological arsenal against deadly diseases.

Ironically, in the midst of these wondrous advances comes a resurgence of interest in alternative medicine. In lieu of today's synthetic preparations, many people are reassessing the use of botanical medications. This recent attention to natural medicines Jefferson would find satisfying. It is the Jeffersonian model of evaluative health care and free thought, individuals taking charge and accepting the responsibility of health maintenance. Dietary habits are also being altered. People are consuming more vegetables and less fatty meats. Vegetables, research is finding, are laden with disease-fighting nutrients. Everything from asparagus to zucchini is being eaten now on a greater scale than at any time over the past several decades. Jefferson would be pleased. Were he alive today, he would encourage this trend towards "garden medicine."

With further confirmation of the health benefits derived from consuming vegetables, the practice will become more popular. More people will decide that dining on increased amounts of vegetables and employing botanical remedies make good sense. It may all become standard practice, and thus will exert great influence on the nation's health.

Thomas Jefferson was the architect of a healthy lifestyle. He enjoyed a life full of enduring accomplishments built upon sound health practices. His occasional bouts with illness demanded flexibility and required an occasional visit from the doctor. These visits were the result of necessity, not hypocrisy. Jefferson was aware of his limitations. When he reached them he sought help. He never stumbled blindly into a course of treatment but rather moved deliberately. He involved himself in the diagnosis and cure of his illnesses. Jefferson was determined to participate in all the stages of his quest to be healthy. This was an integral part of his character: to take charge, to direct events rather than to be directed by them. Control was security.

Jefferson died July 4, 1826, from a combination of old age and the lingering effects of bowel and prostate problems. His physical presence was gone but his example remained, as it does today, a reminder to Americans that it is their duty to succeed in life and prosper in health and happiness. To do so as Jefferson did, Americans must subdue their appetites and control their potential for excess. A few years before he died, Jefferson, extolling his health and peering into the future, wrote to Dr. Benjamin Waterhouse,

> Still. . . I enjoy good health and spirits, and am as industrious a reader as when a student at college. When I contemplate the immense advances in science and discoveries in the arts which have been made within the period of my life, I look forward with confidence to equal advances by the present generation, and have no doubt they will consequently be as much wiser than we have been as we than our fathers were, and they than the burners of witches.[26]

Thomas Jefferson, author of the world's greatest declaration of freedom, who spoke with kings and governed a nation, gazed toward the horizon and saw greatness in those who were to follow. Future generations, he believed with certainty, would transcend human foibles and with wisdom and vigor pursue life, liberty, happiness—and good health.

26 A. Koch and W. Peden, eds., *The Life and Selected Writings of Thomas Jefferson* (New York: Random House, 1993), p. 627.

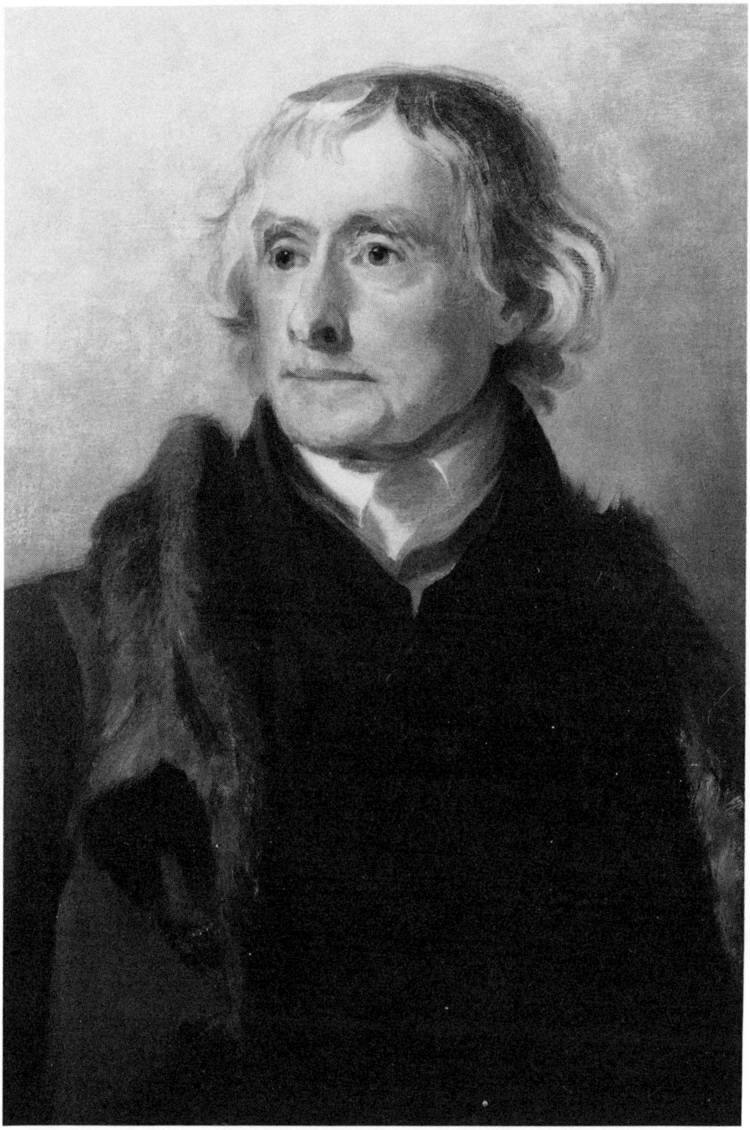

Thomas Jefferson

This bust portrait of Thomas Jefferson hangs in the entrance hall at Monticello. It was copied by Thomas Sulley in 1856 from his original 1821 Life Portrait of Thomas Jefferson, which is at West Point.

Courtesy of the Thomas Jefferson Memorial Foundation; gift of Mr. and Mrs. Carl W. Smith and Mr. and Mrs. T. Eugene Worrel

CHAPTER SEVEN

CONCLUSIONS

A Twentieth-Century Man

THOMAS JEFFERSON'S HEALTH AND MEDICINAL PRACtices are facets of his life that until now have been largely ignored. While many works have touched on his health, none have dealt with it in detail. Nor, have they considered his pharmacological practices or provided many details of his health care habits. This is the first attempt to bring together all three of these topics in some detail.

In the course of researching this work it became evident that, with rare exception, Jefferson kept records of neither problems with his health nor of the medicines used to treat them. If such material exists it has yet to come to light. What information is available can be found in his personal correspondence, letters from family and friends and, at least one physician's fee book.

Clearly, there is much work left to be done to fully uncover the record of Jefferson's health and use of medicine. Currently, thousands of his personal papers are being catalogued and edited at Princeton University. Buried in the myriad of documents may be information that will help to answer many of the remaining questions.

For a man who was obsessed by the smallest details, it seems strange that Jefferson neglected to record the matter of his health. Perhaps he took the same approach to his health that he took to religion, believing them both personal affairs and not appropriate for open discussion. There is a hint of this attitude in portions of his correspondence with Benjamin Rush concerning some of Jefferson's physical problems. And as Paul K. Conkin has noted, "Jefferson had for years argued that religious beliefs were private matters," and, "he consistently refused . . . to state his own. . . ."[1]

While it cannot be proven conclusively that Jefferson used his herbs and plants medicinally, it is almost certain that he cultivated them for that purpose. The evidence available supports this likelihood. Several of Jefferson's herbs had only a single virtue, they were strictly medicinal. Jefferson would have grown them for only one purpose—therapy. The remaining herbs were valuable for their versatility, possessing culinary as well as medicinal qualities. Not only could they medicate, but they were able to season as well, an advantage that would appeal to the utilitarian Jefferson.

Several valuable conclusions can be drawn from this look at Jefferson's health and use of medicines, and go far toward

---

1 Peter S. Onuf, ed., *Jeffersonian Legacies* (Charlottesville, Virginia: University Press of Virginia, 1993), p. 35.

providing a better understanding of Thomas Jefferson, the man. They lend insight into the character and private side of the reticent resident of Monticello.

To begin with, Jefferson could be very like the average man. Like many of his contemporaries he was deeply suspicious of doctors and their treatments. As a consequence, when possible, he doctored himself, as did so many people, with home remedies. In this behavior Jefferson exhibited two common but distinctive American traits—independent thought and action.

With his independence, Jefferson fashioned a style of living and thinking in much the same manner that he constructed Monticello and, like Monticello, the style was uniquely his own. Over time, he diligently devised a lifestyle and thought process based on common sense and reason. Using these two basic elements of judgment, Jefferson was able to live and think with foresight. It was this foresight that fostered development of the health habits that served him so well in his later life.

Admittedly, there are times when Jefferson acted and thought with apparent contradiction. When he was warning against the dangers of using medicines while he used them himself, or suddenly promoting morality over health as a priority, or complaining of faddish and foolish medical treatments and then engaging in some, his true tenets seem to have been preempted to serve some other purpose. It might be tempting to judge his viewpoints as self-serving and transient but he was basically honest in his principles and conduct.

Another finding worth noting is that Jefferson had the courage of his convictions when it came to medicine. Despite contrary examples set by many of his peers, he was willing to stand against the conventional medical wisdom of the day. He cautiously avoided any exertions by doctors to employ heroic medicine against any of his ailments. He did not hesitate to speak out against what he perceived to be the violent and irresponsible treatment of patients who had trustingly placed themselves under a doctor's care. He did so seemingly without concern that it might cost him the connections that he enjoyed with several prominent physicians. His association with them apparently was in spite of, not because of, the fact that they were medical practitioners. Jefferson was a seeker of learning and he obviously felt that these men had things to teach him. He could also have believed that through his association with them he might have some influence in bringing needed change to the field of medicine.

Although Jefferson was cautious about calling in a doctor, he had many friends, such as Benjamin Franklin, who reportedly sought out a physician for any disorder. Jefferson and Franklin did share, however, a peculiar affinity for unusual health habits: Jefferson had his cold water foot baths, Franklin, each morning, read and wrote in the nude.[2] Jefferson's foot baths were perhaps fatuous, but still a far cry from bloodletting, purging and emetics. Jefferson was most often his own man and, with issues such as his health, he took his own counsel.

He did, however, maintain an open mind towards medicine. He was not one to dismiss anything completely. He was amenable, when necessary, to involving a physician in efforts at restoring his health. He might have reluctantly agreed that most doctors had good intentions. However, he would more than likely also have agreed that "the road to Hell is paved with good intentions." Because of this, Jefferson was always ready to exercise his right of final refusal when dealing with doctors and their treatments.

Jefferson was convinced of the value of his health habits. He believed that they held him in good stead and he encour-

---

2 David Freeman Hawke, *Franklin* (New York: Harper & Row, 1976), p. 257.

aged others to emulate them when he had the opportunity. He adhered to the concept of the greatest good for the greatest number. He believed he was onto something beneficial and was eager and willing to share it. Jefferson was nothing, if not confident; in terms of his health practices, he brimmed with self-assurance.

Jefferson's possible opium dependence warrants further study. If in fact such a dependency was present, it would be similar to that of others during his time who innocently found themselves addicted to this potent narcotic. It would not diminish Jefferson's accomplishments any more than the married Benjamin Franklin's flagrant dalliances with other women have devalued his. The addictive potential of opium was simply not understood by most physicians in Jefferson's day; furthermore, opium's unique ability to treat a wide variety of illnesses made it a powerful accessory in medicine's fight against disease. As a result, doctor and patient alike were compelled to ignore, assuming they recognized, any dependence that might have developed.

Perhaps the most pointed finding is that Jefferson, in many facets, was a genuine twentieth-century man. In the first place, by living to the age of eighty-three, he exceeded today's life expectancy for white males by almost a decade. Jefferson would concede that this was owing in part to good luck, but he would also credit his fitness program which very much resembled a contemporary health agenda. His low fat diet, preference for vegetables, abstinence from hard spirits and tobacco, fondness for exercise and love of the outdoors fit perfectly with today's concept of the ideal lifestyle.

His passion for nature and all of her operations would earn him many friends in today's environmental movement. Jefferson understood the need for progress. In fact, he was a proponent of it. But Jefferson would never have sacrificed nature's wonders for an appearance of progress. In his efforts at designing a better plough, developing hardier varieties of seeds and breeding stronger, woollier sheep, he viewed nature as a partner, not an obstruction. Jefferson believed that nature had a *modus operandi* and that man should work with it, not against it.[3] He held nature in the highest esteem and marveled at her creations.

The extensive number of medical works in Jefferson's library attest to his interest in the topic and the attention that he gave it. He could afford more of such books than could the average individual, but his purpose in having them was identical to that of the less affluent. Medical reference volumes were a link with what was known about diseases and treatments. They offered their owners a reservoir of information on the preparation and use of botanical medicines. Medical guides were the emergency rooms of colonial medicine.

Using the herbs in his garden for medicine would place Jefferson in the middle of today's resurgence of interest in botanical remedies. The fascination with natural cures has skyrocketed in recent years. The market for herb and plant medicines is expanding almost daily. People seek natural treatments for everything from weight control to reproductive problems to cancer. Others seek out a myriad of remedies in the hope of enhancing their general health.

It was for similar reasons that Jefferson believed botany to be one of the most valuable sciences. Time has proven him correct. The drugs that have been discovered in plants and the health benefits with which they provide us verify that Jefferson's faith in them was not misplaced. And, the more

---

3 A. Koch and W. Peden, eds., *The Life and Selected Writings of Thomas Jefferson* (New York: Random House, 1993), p. 524.

plants are studied, the more we are made aware of their vast potential.

In keeping with Jefferson's futuristic thinking was his notion of doctor-assisted suicide. He openly supported the dispensing of a drug to terminally ill patients with which they might end their suffering. Only recently has American society begun seriously to discuss such a prospect. This nationwide discussion, fostered by the actions of Dr. Kevorkian, has lately begun to have its effect on the national conscience. Recently, a federal appeals court struck down one state's ban on doctor-assisted suicide. That court declared that the terminally ill have a constitutional right to die with as much dignity and comfort as can be afforded them.

This decision mirrors Jefferson's position of almost two hundred years ago. He held that a person's right to control his own health care implies the right to control the time and manner of death at a time of terminal illness; death is the ultimate personal issue and as such is inviolable. Dignity in death was the goal Thomas Jefferson was advancing with his support of physician-assisted suicide. This makes clear his position that self-determination, in any form, must not be constrained by social mores.

Thomas Jefferson's ideas on health, medicine and dying clearly mark him as a modern man. Although he lived during a more primitive era, his beliefs transcended his place in time and truly made him a man for the ages. There is no reason to suppose that his ideas will not remain as original in the next century as when he developed them, and as they are now.

Jefferson's lifetime was essentially free of illnesses that would have confined him to bed or worse. He tempered his appetites and concentrated on preserving his health. Good health allowed him the joys of family, friends and home. He was totally devoted to his family and freely gave to them his time and possessions. To his friends he was gracious, loyal and a ready source of assistance and support. At Monticello, surrounded by family, called upon by friends and tending his gardens, he found the world a good place to live, with the cares of life within his own control.

Had Thomas Jefferson not guarded his health the history of this nation might very well be different. His contributions to the political, social and cultural development of the young United States might not have occurred. His vision of greatness for America and his trust that Americans will never forget their debt to the patriots of 1776 might never have been sustained by him to be passed on to succeeding generations. Health, good health, was the foundation upon which Jefferson was able to build a legacy for all future Americans.

APPENDIX

Mr. Jefferson's Herbs

SAGE

Early uses—
stays bleeding of wounds, diuretic, helps hoarseness and coughing

Contemporary uses—
as a carminative, a tea for excessive sweating and for nervous disorders

BALM

Early uses—
weak stomach, an electuary, aides digestion

Contemporary uses—
treats feverish colds and headaches and to calm nervous stomachs; helps heal wounds and insect bites

MINT

Early uses—
carminative, poultices, cures nausea

Contemporary uses—
as a carminative and as a refreshing tea

THYME
Early uses—
purges phlegm, and aids shortness of breath; ointment cures warts
Contemporary uses—
used to relieve coughing

LAVENDER
Early uses—
helps cure pains of the head, gargle relieves toothaches
Contemporary uses—
oil used for intestinal distress

MARJORAM
Early uses—
good for colds, obstructions of the spleen; chewed it draws out phlegm
Contemporary uses—
stomach disorders and as a diuretic

CAMOMILE
Early uses—
for agues, sore muscles and pains in the joints
Contemporary uses—
indigestion; appetite stimulant and as an anti-inflammatory

TANSY
Early uses—
carminative, effective against worms and aches in the joints
Contemporary uses—
to expel worms and as an anti-spasmodic

RUE
Early uses—
antidote for poisoning, cholic and weaknesses of the bowels
Contemporary uses—
anti-spasmodic and cough suppressant

WORMWOOD
Early uses—
for weakness of the stomach and gout

Contemporary uses—
anthelmintic and as an emmenagogue

SOUTHERNWOOD
Early uses—
treatment for worms, helps cramps and convulsions
Contemporary uses—
intestinal worms and as an antiseptic

ROSEMARY
Early uses—
helps treat a cold, excellent carminative, comforts the stomach
Contemporary uses—
intestinal worms and as an antiseptic

HYSSOP
Early uses—
treat quinsy (throat swelling), helps cure toothaches
Contemporary uses—
coughs, hoarseness and sore throat

PERIWINKLE
Early uses—
infusion stays the menses, prevents bleeding at the mouth and nose
Contemporary uses—
hemostatic and reduces blood pressure

MARSHMALLOW
Early uses—
Produces a mucilage for ointments and poultices for inflammations; treats irritated eyes
Contemporary uses—
gargle for sore throat and a mucilage to soothe the skin

BEARGRASS
Early uses—
undetermined
Contemporary uses—
none known

Bibliography

Ammon, Harry. *James Monroe—The Quest for National Identity.* New York: McGraw-Hill Book Company, 1971.

Anderson, Frank J. *An Illustrated History of the Herbals.* New York: Columbia University Press, 1977.

Bear, James A., Jr., and Gordon Jones, MD. *Thomas Jefferson and His Health.* Unpublished monograph, Monticello Research Center.

——— and Lucia C. Stanton, eds. *Jefferson's Memorandum Books: Accounts, with Legal Records and Miscellany, 1767–1826.* Princeton, New Jersey: Princeton University Press, forthcoming.

Betts, Edwin Morris, ed. *Thomas Jefferson's Garden Book: 1766–1824.* Lancaster, Pennsylvania: Lancaster Press, Inc., 1944.

———, ed. *Thomas Jefferson's Farm Book.* Princeton, New Jersey: Princeton University Press, 1953.

——— and James Adam Bear, Jr., eds. *The Family Letters of Thomas Jefferson.* Columbia, Missouri: University of Missouri Press, 1966.

——— and Hazlehurst B. Perkins. *Thomas Jefferson's Flower Garden at Monticello.* Charlottesville, Virginia: University of Virginia Press, 1986.

Bishop, Arthur, ed. *Thomas Jefferson, 1743–1826.* Dobbs Ferry, New York: Oceana Publications, Inc., 1971.

Blanton, Wyndham B. *Medicine in the Seventeenth Century.* Richmond, Virginia: The William Byrd Press, Inc., 1930.

———. *Medicine in the Eighteenth Century.* Richmond, Virginia: Garrett & Massie, Incorporated, 1931.

Boorstin, Daniel J. *The Americans: The Colonial Experience.* New York: Vintage Books, 1958.

Boyd, Julian P., ed. *The Papers of Thomas Jefferson.* 25 vols. Princeton, New Jersey: Princeton University Press, 1950.

Boykin, Edward. *To the Boys and Girls.* New York: Funk & Wagnalls Company, Inc., 1964.

Brodie, Fawn M. *Thomas Jefferson—An Intimate History.* New York: W.W. Norton and Company, Inc., 1974.

Butterfield, L. H., ed. *Diary and Autiobiography of John Adams.* 4 vols. Cambridge, Massachusetts: The Belknap Press of Harvard University, 1961.

Capps, Benjamin. *The Indians.* New York: Time-Life Books, 1973.

Clark, Ronald W. *Benjamin Franklin.* New York: Random House, 1983.

Clinton, Catherine. *The Plantation Mistress.* New York: Pantheon Books, 1982.

Colonial Dames of America. *Herbs and Herb Lore of Colonial America.* New York: Dover Publications, Inc., 1995.

Cullen, William. *A Treatise of the Materia Medica.* Edinburgh: publisher unknown, 1789.

Culpeper, Nicholas. *Culpeper's Complete Herbal.* London: W. Foulsham & Company, Ltd., unknown.

de Treville, Lawrence R., III. *Jefferson and Wine: Model of Moderation.* The Plains, Virginia: The Vinifera Wine Growers Association, Inc., 1989.

Dorsey, John M., MD, ed. *The Jefferson-Dunglison Letters.* Charlottesville, Virginia: University of Virginia Press, 1960.

Duncan, Andrew. *The Edinburgh New Dispensatory.* Philadelphia: T. Dobson, 1791.

Dwyer, James and David Rattray, eds., et-al. *Magic and Medicine of Plants.* Pleasantville, New York: The Readers Digest Association, Inc., 1993.

Flexner, James Thomas. *Washington—The Indispensable Man.* Boston: Little, Brown and Company, 1969.

Foley, J. P., ed. *The Jefferson Cyclopedia.* 2 vols. New York: Russell and Russell, 1967.

Fuller, Thomas. *Pharmacopoeia Extemporanea.* London: B. Walford, 1740.

Gill, Harold B., Jr. *The Apothecary in Colonial Virginia.* Williamsburg, Virginia: The Colonial Williamsburg Foundation, 1972.

Griggs, Barbara. *Green Pharmacy.* Rochester, Vermont: Healing Arts Press, 1991.

Hawke, David Freeman. *Franklin.* New York: Harper and Row, 1976.

Harrison, Maureen and Steve Bilbert, eds. *Thomas Jefferson: Word for Word.* LaJolla, Calofornia: Excellent Books, 1993.

Hughes, Thomas P. *Medicine in Virginia, 1607–1699.* Historical booklet number 21. Williamsburg, Virginia: Virginia 350th Anniversary Celebration Corporation, 1957.

Irving, Washington. *George Washington: A Biography.* New York: De Capo Press, 1994.

Jackson, Donald. *A Year at Monticello—1795.* Golden, Colorado: Fulcrum, Inc., 1989.

Josephy, Alvin M., Jr., ed. *The American Heritage Book of Indians.* New York: American Heritage Publishing Company, Inc./Bonanza Books, 1982.

Ketcham, Ralph. *James Madison: A Biography.* New York: The Macmillan Company, 1971.

Kimball, Marie. *Thomas Jefferson's Cookbook.* Richmond, Virginia: Garrett & Massie, Inc., 1938.

Koch, Adrienne and William Peden, eds. *The Life and Selected Writings of Thomas Jefferson.* New York: The Modern Library, 1944.

Kowalchik, Claire and William H. Hylton, eds. *Illustrated Encyclopedia of Herbs.* Emmaus, Pennsylvania: Rodale Press, 1987.

Lewis, Walter H. *Medical Botany.* New York: John Wiley & Sons, 1977.

McIntyre, Anne. *Herbs for Common Ailments.* New York: Simon & Schuster, Inc., 1992.

Malone, Dumas. *Jefferson and His Time.* 5 vols. Boston: Little, Brown and Company, 1948.

Marquis, Mary. *A Short Synopsis of the Uses of Medicinal Plants—Herbs—From Past to Present.* Unpublished paper, 1995.

——— and Lynn M. Richmond. *Objects for the Garden: Useful Plants From Jefferson's Time.* published by the authors, 1994.

Miller, Charles A. *Jefferson and Nature.* Baltimore, Maryland: The Johns Hopkins University Press, 1988.

Morris, Richard B. and Jeffrey B. Morris, eds. *Encyclopedia of American History.* New York: Harper & Row, 1976.

Numbus, Ronald L. and Todd L. Savitt, eds. *Science and Medicine in the Old South.* Baton Rouge, Louisiana: Louisiana State University Press, 1989.

Peterson, Merrill D. *Thomas Jefferson: Writings.* New York: The Library of America, 1984.

———, ed. *Visitors to Monticello.* Charlottesville, Virginia: University of Virginia Press, 1989.

Randall, Henry S. *The Life of Thomas Jefferson.* 3 vols. New York: Derby & Jackson, 1858.

Randolph, Sarah N. *The Domestic Life of Thomas Jefferson.* Cambridge, Massachusetts: University Press, 1939.

Salmon, William. *Pharmacopoeia Londinensis.* London: publisher unknown, 1682.

Savitt, Todd L. *Medicine and Slavery.* Urbana, Illinois: University of Illinois Press, 1978.

———. *Fevers, Agues and Cures.* Richmond, Virginia: Virginia Historical Society, 1990.

Sawvel, Franklin B., ed. *The Anas of Thomas Jefferson.* New York: De Capo Press, 1970.

Sowerby, E. Millicent. *Catalogue of the Library of Thomas Jefferson.* 5 vols. Washington, D.C.: The Library of Congress, 1952.

Smith, Richard Norton. *Patriarch.* Boston: Houghton Mifflin Company, 1993.

Steinberg, Alfred. *John Marshall.* New York: G. P. Putnam's Sons, 1962.

Taylor, Norman. *Plant Drugs that Changed the World.* New York: Dodd, Mead & Company, 1965.

Tucker, George. *The Life of Thomas Jefferson.* Carey, Lea & Blanchard, 1837.

Viola, Herman J. and Carolyn Margolis. *Seeds of Change.* Washington, D.C.: Smithsonian Institution Press, 1991.

Williamsburg Craft Series. *The Apothecary in Eighteenth Century Williamsburg.* 1987.

Zimmerman, David R. *The Essential Guide to Nonprescription Drugs.* New York: Harper and Row, 1983.

Index

A

acetylsalicylic acid
See aspirin
acrimony, 58
Adams, John, 5, 19, 68
agues, 13, 52, 57, 110
Albany Indians
See Indians, Albany
Althaea officinalis
See marshmallow
American Indians
See Indians
anthelmintic, 57, 111
Anthemis nobilis
See chamomile
apothecary shops, 39
apples, 71
Artemisia abrotanum
See southernwood
Artemisia absinthium
See wormwood
aspirin, 92
asthma, 8
astringents, 15, 37, 43, 44, 78

B

balm, vi, 14, 40, 49, 52, 53, 109
Bankhead, Anne Cary Randolph, 32, 70
basil, 14
baths, mineral, 26, 27, 30, 31
Baynard, Edward, 73
beans, 71, 93
Bear, James A., Jr., 4, 5, 26, 30, 31, 33, 34, 43, 47, 48, 53, 55, 58, 61, 62, 70, 75, 77, 78, 80, 82, 89, 91, 93
beargrass, 40, 58, 111
Bellini, Charles, 49
Betts, Edwin Morris, 4, 5, 15, 16, 26, 33, 34, 39, 40, 43, 44, 47, 48, 53, 55, 70, 71, 75, 76, 77, 78, 80, 91, 93
Beverley, Robert, 24
bladder senna, 44
bleeding, 1, 5, 9, 17, 18, 22, 29, 51, 52, 58, 90, 104, 109, 111
blue flag, 8
botany, 45, 92, 106
bougie, 32
bowel, 13, 29, 31, 35, 36, 37, 44, 53, 54, 56, 62, 80, 81, 90, 98, 110
Brodie, Fawn, 4
Brown, Robert, Dr., 48
Brown, Samuel, Dr., 46, 50
Byrd, William, 16, 43

C

Cabell, William, 16
calomel, 28, 29, 30, 34, 56, 63, 88
camphor, 61
Capsicum
See pepper
Carr, Peter, 74, 75, 88, 89
Catanzariti, John, 5
cayenne pepper
See pepper
chamomile, vi, 13, 14, 15, 40, 41, 51, 56
cholera, 3
codeine, 36, 92
cold, common, vii, viii, 2, 3, 40, 45, 68, 69, 73, 80, 81, 82, 104, 109, 110, 111
College of William and Mary, 49

"constipating purge", 43
Cooper, Thomas, Dr., 18, 45
corn salve, 63
Creek Indians
    See Indians, Creek
cucumber, 70, 71
Cullen, William, 41, 52, 53, 56, 57
Culpeper, Nicholas, 13, 14, 15, 40, 41, 43, 44, 47, 48, 52, 54, 55, 57, 58
cupping, 13

D

dandelion, 13, 16
dandruff, 8
Datura-Stramomium
    See James-Town weed
Declaration of Independence, vii, 17, 37, 87
diarrhea, 3, 13, 30, 31, 32, 34, 36, 37, 43, 44, 50, 53, 61, 69, 79, 80, 81, 82, 89
diet, 2, 5, 67, 69, 71, 72, 79, 81, 83, 90, 105
digitalis, 92
Dioscorea, 92
diphtheria, 3, 12, 14, 81
Duncan, Andrew, 41, 54, 55
Dunglison, Robley, Dr., vi, 18, 21, 25, 26, 29, 31, 32, 33, 34, 35, 36, 37, 43, 44, 50, 61, 86, 90, 91, 95

E

Edinburgh New Dispensatory, The, 41, 54, 55
emetics, 1, 8, 12, 16, 22, 29, 41, 88, 104
endive, 70
England, 2, 54, 90
    London, 14, 15, 21, 39, 40, 43, 44, 48, 54, 55, 56, 57, 58
Eppes, Francis Wayles, 26, 78, 94
Eppes, Mary Jefferson, 78, 94
Euphorbia Ipecacuanhae
    See ipecac
exercise, 2, 5, 18, 67, 69, 73–76, 79, 81, 83, 87, 90, 94, 95, 104, 105

F

faddish medical treatments, 103
fever, 12, 13, 27, 30, 52, 53, 62, 78, 80, 81, 109
    ague, 13, 27, 52, 57, 110
    intermittent, 12, 52
    slow, 12
    yellow, 27, 81
flux, 13, 15
foxglove, 92
France, 26, 30, 57
    Aix-en-Provence, 26
    Paris, 26, 74, 93
Franklin, Benjamin, 5, 26, 42, 104, 105
Fry, Henry, 81
Fuller, Thomas, 41

G

Garden Book, 28, 39, 43, 44, 59, 70, 71, 76
gardening, 35, 71, 76, 77
General Therapeutics and Materia Medica, 35, 37, 43
gerkin, 71
Gilmer, George, Jr., 25, 50
ginseng, 14
"God's own medicine", 61
Greek, 95
gum Arabic, 63

H

headaches, vii, viii, 3, 30, 55, 56, 58, 62, 63, 79, 80, 82, 109
Hemings, Sally, 4, 88
heroic medicine, 19, 23, 29, 90, 103
Hill, John, Sir, 73
Horner, Gustavus, Dr., 45, 50
horseback riding, 35, 74, 76, 81
hyssop, vi, 14, 40, 49, 58, 111

I

immigrants
    German, 11
    Scotch, 11
    Scotch-Irish, 11
Indian physic, 16

Indians, 7, 8, 9, 11, 16
  Albany, 8
  Creek, 8
  Meskwakis, 8
  Ojibwa, 8
  Penobscots, 8
infusions, 41, 42, 111
intermittents, 12, 29, 52
ipecac, 13, 16

J

jalap, 28, 34
James-Town weed, 46
Jefferson, Randolph, 71
Jefferson, Thomas, vi, vii, viii, 1, 2, 3, 4, 5, 15, 16, 17, 18, 19, 20, 21, 22, 23, 25, 26, 27, 28, 29, 30, 31, 32, 33, 34, 35, 36, 37, 39, 40, 41, 42, 43, 44, 45, 46, 47, 48, 49, 50, 51, 52, 53, 54, 55, 56, 57, 58, 59, 60, 61, 62, 63, 64, 65, 67, 68, 69, 70, 71, 72, 73, 74, 75, 76, 77, 78, 79, 80, 81, 82, 83, 84, 85, 86, 87, 88, 89, 90, 91, 92, 93, 94, 95, 96, 97, 98, 99, 101, 102, 103, 104, 105, 106, 107, 108
Jefferson's medicine box, 63, 64
Jeffersonia diphylla, 45
Jesuits bark
  See quinine
Jones, Gordon, M.D., 30, 82

K

Kevorkian, Jack, Dr., 46, 107
Koch, Adrienne, 4, 22, 23, 34, 46, 49, 68, 69, 72, 73, 74, 75, 77, 78, 79, 80, 82, 85, 87, 88, 94, 98, 106
Koscuisko, Thaddeus, 94

L

laudanum, 28, 32, 35–37, 61, 62
Lavandula spica
  See lavender
lavender, vi, 14, 15, 40, 41, 54, 55, 56, 110
laxative, 37, 44
lettuce, 70
Lewis and Clark expedition, 93
Lewis, Walter, 16, 93
lifestyle, 2, 19, 36, 76, 79, 94, 97, 103, 105
liniment, 48
lobelia, 14, 41, 43

M

Madeira
  See wine
magnesia, 28, 32, 37
malaria, 2, 3, 12, 13, 14, 30, 52
Malone, Dumas, 4, 45, 59, 69, 77, 86, 89
marjoram, vi, 40, 51, 110
Marjorana hortensis
  See marjoram
Marshall, John, 19
marshmallow, vi, 40, 58, 111
Maryland, Baltimore, 78
Massachusetts, 19, 31, 49, 67, 69, 74, 75, 76, 78, 79
materia medica, 3, vii, 8, 40, 50
meat, 18, 69, 72, 97
medicine box
  See Jefferson's medicine box
Melissa officinalis
  See balm
Mentha piperita
  See mint
mercury, 25, 29, 30, 34
Meskwakis
  See Indians, Meskwakis
Miller, John Chester, 4
mineral baths
  See baths, mineral
mint, vi, 8, 40, 51, 53, 57, 109, 111
Mitchell, John, Dr., 42
Monticello, vi, vii, ix, 4, 5, 15, 26, 28, 30, 31, 32, 34, 36, 39, 41, 43, 44, 46, 47, 50, 51, 53, 56, 57, 58, 59, 60, 61, 64, 68, 69, 70, 71, 76, 78, 83, 89, 91, 92, 99, 103, 108
morphine, 36, 92
mosquito, anopheles, 12
Mount Vernon, 19
Munford, William Green, 22

N

nausea, 8, 109
Neuville, Monsieur de, 79
New Hampshire, 41
Notes on the State of Virginia, 16, 22

O

Ohio, 71
Ojibwa
See Indians, Ojibwa
opium, 29, 35, 36, 61, 92, 105
opium dependence, 35, 105

P

Palma christi
See ricinus
paregoric, 61
peaches, 71
Peale, Charles Willson, 73, 93
"periodical headaches", 55, 62, 65, 80
Peden, William, 4, 22, 23, 34, 46, 49, 68, 69, 72, 73, 74, 75, 77, 78, 79, 80, 82, 85, 87, 88, 94, 98, 106
Pedro Ximenes
See wine
Pennsylvania, Philadelphia, 10, 17, 54, 55, 70, 80, 92, 93
Penobscots
See Indians, Penobscots
pepper, 47, 48, 53
peristaltic action, 35
periwinkle, vi, 15, 40, 58, 111
Peruvian Bark
See quinine
Peterson, Merrill, 4, 22
physic, 9, 16, 40, 63
physician-assisted suicide, 46, 107
placebo effect, 23
pneumonia, 81
Poplar Forest, 49
poppy, 92
Princeton University, 102
prostate, 32, 98
purges, 1, 5, 42, 43, 44, 54, 58, 110
putrid sore throat, 12, 13

Q

quinine, 12, 28, 30
Quinsy, rotten, 12, 13, 14

R

rabies, 14
Randall, Henry, 4, 74
Randolph, Ellen Wayles, 53
Randolph, Martha Jefferson, 36, 59
Randolph, Sarah Jefferson, 4, 74, 76
Randolph, Thomas Jefferson, 31, 70, 74, 78
Randolph, Thomas Mann, 59, 60, 68
Randolph, Thomas Mann, Jr., 85
Rheum rhaponticum
See rhubarb
Rheum undulatum
See rhubarb
rheumatism, 3, 26, 27, 47, 48
rhubarb, 14, 28, 32, 37, 43, 44
ricinus, 16
Ricketson, Shadrach, 73
Riverius, Lazarus, 41
Rosemarinus officinalis
See rosemary
rosemary, vi, 40, 49, 50, 51, 58, 111
rue, vi, 8, 14, 15, 29, 40, 49, 51, 56, 57, 75, 90, 103, 110
running, 57, 62, 76
Rush's Thunderbolts, 34
Rush, Benjamin, Dr., 17, 18, 25, 30, 31, 34, 43, 48, 49, 50, 53, 61, 79, 80, 87, 89, 102
Ruta graveolens
See rue

S

sage, vi, 36, 40, 41, 42, 50, 51, 52, 53, 65, 79, 109
salad (or sallad), 44, 59, 70
sallad oil, 70
Salmon, William, 41, 56, 58
Salvia officinalis
See sage
sassafras, 14, 19
senna, 13, 43, 44
sesame, 44

Sesamum trifoliatum
See sesame
Short, William, 34, 83
skunk cabbage, 8
slaves, vii, 4, 37, 88
smallpox, 3
Smith, John, 9
snake-root, 16
soaproot, 8
southernwood, vi, 15, 16, 40, 49, 51, 57, 111
Sowerby, E. Millicent, 41, 45, 73, 81
Stanton, Lucia C., ix, 5, 62
steroids, 92
stress, 27, 32, 36, 47, 59, 60, 80, 81, 110
sudorific, 52
sulphur, 30
swimming, 76
Sydenham, Thomas, Dr., 81
Syracuse
See wine

T

Tanacetum vulgare
See tansy
tansy, vi, 15, 40, 49, 51, 56, 110
Taylor, John, 44
Thomas, Robert, 50, 60
Thomson, Samuel, 41, 43
Thouin, Andre, 93
thyme, vi, 40, 41, 51, 54, 110
Thymus vulgaris
See thyme
tobacco, 5, 18, 19, 67, 69, 76, 77, 81, 83, 105
tonic, 8, 11
tuberculosis, 82
twentieth-century man, 105
typhoid, 12, 13, 14, 81

U

University of Virginia, 21, 31, 33, 71, 73, 77, 90, 91
University of Virginia School of Medicine, 33, 91
Utley, Vine, Dr., 69, 82

V

vegetables, 13, 18, 29, 42, 69, 70, 71, 72, 97, 105
Vinca minor
See periwinkle
Virginia, 7, 9, 10, 11, 12, 15, 16, 24, 31, 41, 42, 48, 52, 73, 81
House of Burgesses, 82
Madison County, 81
Richmond, 48
Urbanna, 42
Warm Springs, 26, 31
Williamsburg, 39
vis medicatrix naturae, 22, 42

W

Washington, George, 5, 17, 19, 42, 88, 94
water, 2, 13, 19, 23, 26, 27, 31, 45, 56, 61, 62, 72, 73, 79, 80, 81, 82, 104
Waterhouse, Benjamin, Dr., 83, 98
Wharton, Thomas, Dr., 39, 40
Wheaton, Henry, Dr., 81
white vitriol, 61
wild mint, 8
wine, 15, 18, 62, 77–79
Wistar, Caspar, Dr., 22, 23, 96
wormwood, vi, 15, 40, 49, 51, 57, 110
Worthington, Thomas, 71

Y

Yucca filamentosa
See beargrass

This book was designed and typeset by AAH Graphics, Inc., Fort Valley, Virginia.

The text type is New Caledonia, based on W.A. Dwiggins's 1938 Caledonia, itself a modernized version of Scotch Roman from the English punchcutter Richard Austin, who introduced it around 1805, and which was first imported into the United States in 1837 by the Boston printer Samuel L. Dickenson.

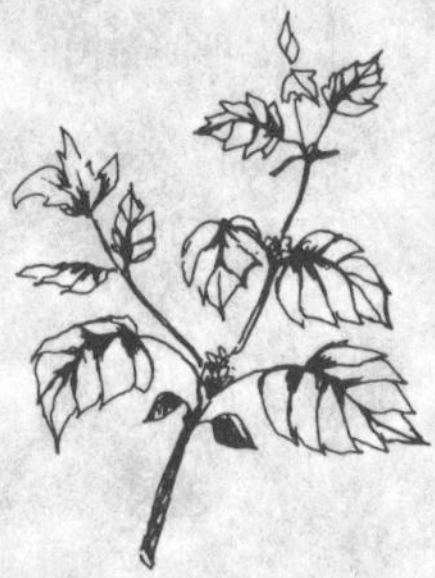

Melissa officinalis

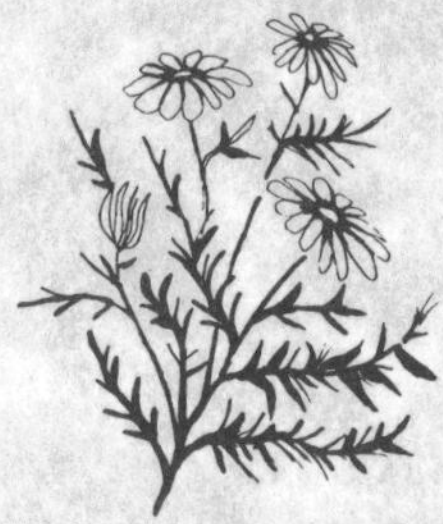

Anthemis nobilis

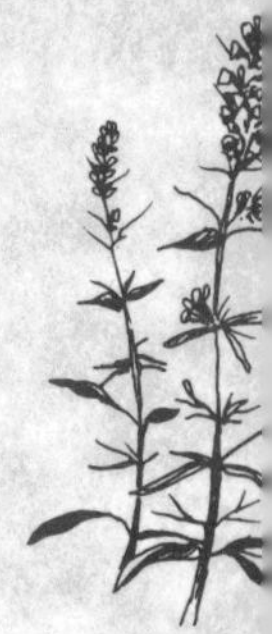

Hyssopus offic

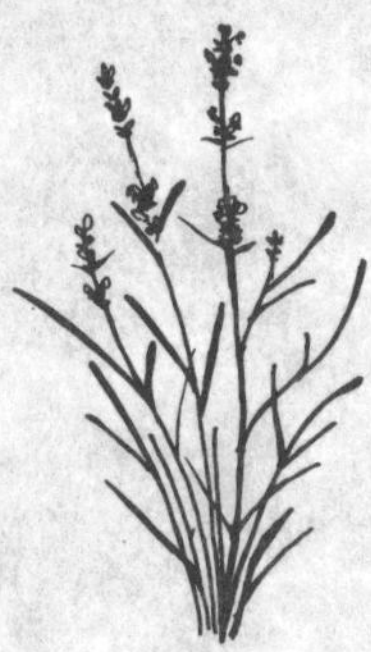

Lavandula spica

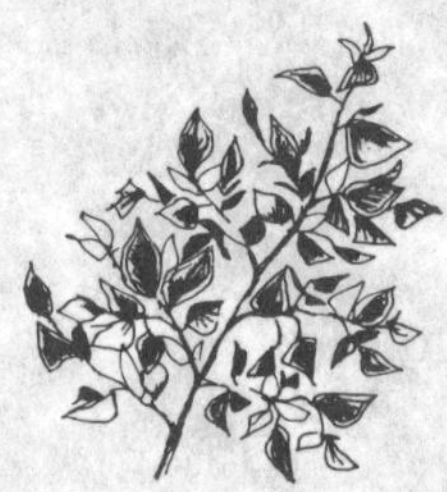

Marjorana hortensis

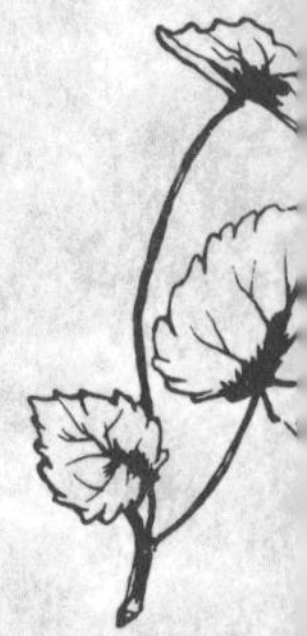

Althaea offic

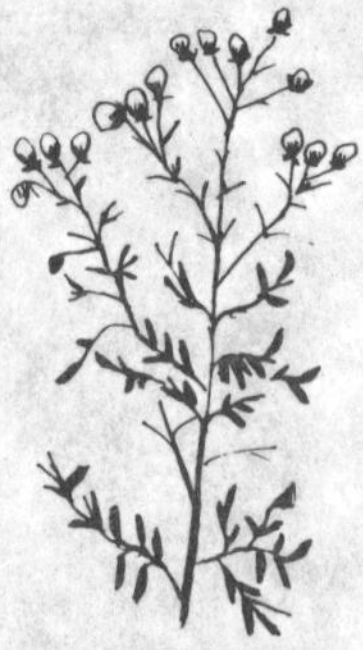

Ruta graveolens

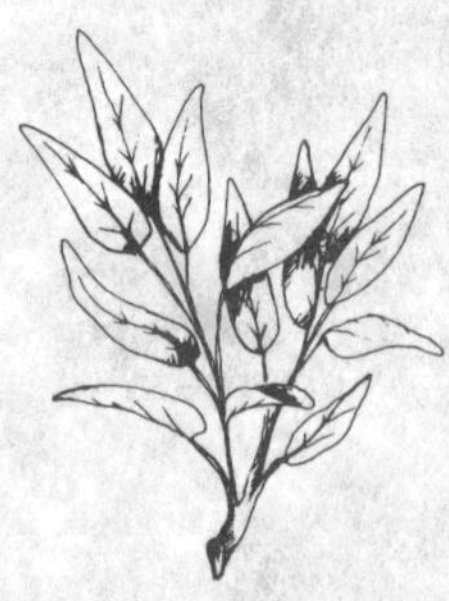

Salvia officinalis

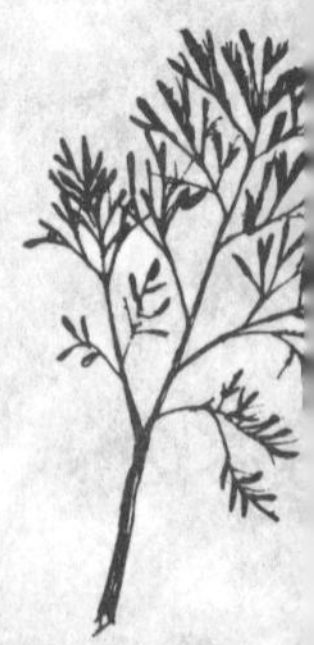

Artemisi abrotanu